STAYING THIN

BY
DR. ROBERT LINN

ZEBRA BOOKS
KENSINGTON PUBLISHING CORP.

ZEBRA BOOKS

are published by

KENSINGTON PUBLISHING CORP.
475 Park Avenue South
New York, N.Y. 10016

Published by arrangement with G. P. Putnam's Sons

Printed in the United States of America

Acknowledgments

Very seldom is a book the product of one person. Others, through encouragement and advice contribute to making something work. My effort here is no exception. A very important part of this book was due to the untiring effort of Ms. Judy Foldes. I must acknowledge a special thanks to her. Above all, thanks to my collaborator, Paulette Cooper.

And then, of course, there are other friends and colleagues who in one way or another make this book possible. To all, perhaps, the best way to put it is simply: Thank you.

To Laurie, Danny and Ricky

Contents

1
Food
Is a
Four-letter Word

Food. The availability of it in our society is overpowering. Supermarkets are Arabian bazaars crammed with every imaginable variety. Temptation lurks in every aisle. And those who try to escape find the streets outside lined with fast food emporia, offering instant gratification to the hit-and-run eater.

Everything seems to tip the scales in favor of being overweight. We—and that no doubt means you—spend more and more time in sedentary positions. Perhaps you sit home night after night, reading a book or watching television—which means food commercials—for hours on end. Or you sit in an office all day, thinking about, dreaming about, munching upon—food. Even when you move from place to place, you sit in your car, being subjected to more food commercials on the radio.

No wonder it's close to impossible to control yourself under such circumstances. But if you are already a compulsive overeater, then even without these constant external reminders, food has come to dominate your life. Do you call a friend and say "Come on over for a nice long chat"? Nonsense. It's far more likely to be "come on over for coffee, or cake, or drinks." Even without the social aspect of food, when you are alone you see an ad for potato chips on television, pass a pizza parlor on the street, or watch a delectable dessert being served at the next restaurant table, and you are off and eating.

The years go by and you find it harder and harder to pass the refrigerator without grabbing a snack. To get through an afternoon's work without a pause that refreshes. Or to get through a long lonely evening without a snack for companionship.

No wonder the battle against fat has turned into an all-out war. And that you so often lose the fray. The heavy artillery is on the enemy's side. All you've got going for you is reduced self-control—and an expanding waistline.

Not surprisingly, there is a whole pharmacopoeia of weight loss programs to deal with our national obsession. One diet achieves instant popularity, only to be rapidly succeeded by another new miracle cure. And actually, many of these diets *do* work their magic. For a while.

But most dieters quickly get caught in a vicious cycle, rapidly regaining those wretched pounds they struggled so hard to lose. And then you are off and at it again. Back to the *new* diet that supposedly makes all other methods obsolete and unnecessary.

And the new diet does work for a while, because the variety and excitement it provides gives you the momentum to control yourself. Temporarily. But then you begin to feel the same old thing—hunger, or rather craving (they are two different things as you'll learn), plus boredom when the new method becomes the old.

And soon you're overeating again.

THERE'S NOTHING JOLLY ABOUT BEING FAT

It's ironic that while there's food every place you turn, being overweight is taboo in our culture. We encourage people to indulge and then punish them for doing so. It hardly seems fair.

It wasn't always that way. In years past, those people who had a "little meat on their bones" were thought the most attractive and sexually desirable. To be called "pleasingly plump" was considered a compliment. And it isn't so long ago that a woman might have been delighted to be described as "fair, fat, and forty."

Fat chance that would please her now. Thin is In. Models, movie stars, TV personalities, the "beautiful people," and other objects of our ephemeral adulation bear no physical resemblance to the rotund Rubens models who were once con-

11

sidered the prototype of beauty. And this goes for you men as well as for women. Have you ever seen a picture of a Marlboro man who looks too fat to get on his horse?

But our admiration of thin people—and our revulsion toward fat—is based on more than just external factors. Fatties turn people off for reasons that are more than skin deep. Others make negative moral judgments about them, too.

Deep down, many of us have a tendency to think less of fatties as people because unconsciously, we construe their circumference as the outer proof of their inner lack of self-control. And you'd better believe that others have thought this way of you if, in the past, you let yourself get really fat, you were showing others that you didn't really care about yourself. And if *you* didn't care, you probably didn't get the respect from others that you wanted or deserved. That makes sense, too. If *you* don't think well of yourself, how can you expect others to hold you in high esteem?

The truth is that deep down, most people find fat people repulsive at worst, pathetic at best. Just as food has dominated fat people's lives, their fat has dominated other people's perception of them. No matter what attributes rotund people have, it's their fat that others are likely to remember.

Elvis Presley is a perfect (and pathetic) example. He proved that fat people not only have to live with their corpulence, but that's often how they're remembered after they die. What color eyes did he have? How tall was he? Was he overweight? Ah, yes. People always notice and remember that about someone, even long after they're gone. Many of Judy Garland's most loyal fans remember her final overweight years more vividly than they recall the sweet little thin girl in *The Wizard of Oz*. Whatever fat people have to offer, it's the memory of their overweight that seems to last through thick and thin.

But people don't have to be dead or famous for their fat to stand out. How often have you heard overweight friends discussed where their weight hasn't cropped up in an unflattering or derogatory way? "What a nice guy. It's such a shame that—" Or "she has such a pretty face. If only—," or "she has so much to offer. Why do you suppose she let herself—" And the fact that you've heard it so often is why you were able to fill the rest of those sentences in now.

In addition, when "straight" people see people who are fat, they often unconsciously conjure up an image of how they got to be that way, of all the *gorging* those people must have done. And it's not a pretty picture. Obese people may have exquisite table manners, but the world tends to view them as the worst kind of gluttons. An unkinder word—but one that is frequently applied—is, plainly put, a pig.

Consider, for example, Henry VIII. When he was young, he was a remarkably handsome man who wrote poetry and music. But who has ever heard anything about his lean years? The image his name evokes today is that of a grotesquely fat man not using his hands creatively but ripping a roast chicken apart with them.

Since fat has a negative significance in most people's minds, and they have drawn certain unfavorable conclusions about the obese, fat people are often discriminated against professionally as well as socially. They don't get jobs as easily as their thinner counterparts. They're less likely to hold on to them (unless they go on a diet), and they tend not to be promoted as rapidly as those with lean and hungry looks.

Has it happened to you? If so, you had better realize that it may have been the least of your problems. Obesity does more than just make you unattractive to other people and hamper your chances for career advancement. It can kill you long before your time. And even when it doesn't cause death, it can virtually cripple you, help cause high blood pressure, heart disease, diabetes, and a host of other ills.

There's a word that criminologists use to describe the failure of criminals to respond to punishment, rehabilitation, or any attempts to cure them of their baser tendencies. Recidivism. The literal meaning of the word is "relapse," a slipping back or losing of gained ground.

You don't have to be a criminal to be a recidivist. You can just be like most dieters. No matter how hard they work not to succumb to the temptations of "illegal" food, no matter how many odious pounds they manage to shed, no matter how many compliments they receive or how much success they attain, after a while, they almost invariably have a relapse.

The Stay Thin method was developed to help you avoid recidivism; to help you live in the world with a permanently thin figure, a healthy body, and a positive self image.

So forget forever the notion of the "jolly fat man." (The only time that person is ever welcome is at Christmas.) Focus instead on the far more accurate picture of the fat person seen as unattractive and thought of as out of control, not to mention being unappreciated, underpaid, and unhealthy. That certainly is far from jolly. What the fat person really is is a recidivist peering out from behind the bars of a self-created prison.

It doesn't ever have to happen to you again. This time you can forget about all those diets, toss away all those pills, and finally Stay Thin forever.

2
How
the Stay Thin Method
Was Developed

WHY YOUR DIETS FAILED

Every hour, every day, in almost every home in America, billions of pounds are being attacked by millions of frustrated people. On the side, most of these people *will* manage to win the immediate battle—if it means enough to them to work diligently at it and suffer long and hard for it. Yet, unhappily, most of them will ultimately lose the War of Weight.

That's because most dieters end up continually gaining and losing weight, suffering from what is aptly and commonly known as the yo-yo syndrome. Up and down, back and forth they go—like hardened criminals going in and out of jail—from svelte to flabby, from fat to firm, sometimes as often as four or five times in a year.

Win. Lose. Win. Lose. The fight goes on. And on. And on.

After many years of this, the weight-losers no longer feel like winners. Not when they realize that they will soon be going through it all again. So there comes a time when, knowing full well that they will only be knocked down again, they no longer have the strength (or the will) to reenter the arena. During certain bouts, it's almost a relief to go down for the final count. Let the pounds return again. The discouraged dieters finally throw in the towel. "Oh God, I worked so hard," they sigh. "I really really tried."

And it's true, too. They *were* persistent. They made every imaginable sacrifice. Time and time again, they said goodbye to goodies. They swore off all the comforting candies, and the tantalizing tempters like pizza and cocktail nuts. They cut out drinking; they gave up picnics and hot lunches; they starved themselves at parties; they carried little baggies of oil-free tuna fish to dinner parties, and bored their friends with calorie-counting conversation and gram-measuring devices. Oh, how virtuous they were.

But as things turned out, it wasn't forever. The pounds crept in, the flab slipped back. It was so unfair, too, since, after all, they had proved repeatedly that they did indeed have the willpower they needed to lose weight. They had paid their dues. They had earned their rest. Yet it was always fat that was the final victor: the undisputed champion!

* * *

By now, you've probably already learned firsthand that most diets *can* help you achieve the dramatic weight losses you seek, but that they almost invariably leave you without the resources necessary to maintain that weight loss for any significant period. All that work seems worthless. It's almost as if you hadn't really lost those pounds—just temporarily misplaced them. And unfortunately, you later found them again.

That's why you need the Stay Thin approach. This time you will at last be able to control your compulsive eating—will never have to go on another diet—because you'll learn to control the very drives that created your compulsive behavior. You will learn how to reexamine your attitudes and your habits and then break down the negative patterns of behavior and thinking that made you a food junkie in the first place.

That's right. You're going to break down—and lose *forever*—the part of you that made you get fat again every time you dieted successfully. You're going to eradicate the unwanted thoughts and stimuli that over and over again lead you to self-destructive eating—often at the very moment of triumph.

And in their place, there's going to be another you. Not just a new slim-for-a-while you, but a life-long pleased-as-punch-with-yourself slim new you forever. A you who will be comfortably "just right" for the rest of your life.

Without having to work as hard as you did on some of your diets, you will become a person who not only will be thin, but more importantly, can *stay* thin. (I'm assuming that most readers of this book are now either at their goal weight, or within twenty pounds of it. If you're, say, fifty pounds off, you still have some hard work ahead of you. But this book can help you too.)

Now, the kind of complete change I'm talking about can't be focused solely in your mouth and your stomach. You've most likely tried that route before with a multitude of diets, and ultimately, you probably failed.

That's because Staying Thin is not simply a matter of what you eat. Indeed, you will see that it is not what you eat but *how* you eat, and even more important, how you *think* that can make you finally succeed in Staying Thin.

Obviously, this is not Another Diet. Instead, you're about to undertake a complete make-over, a transition from one way of living and thinking to another.

Relax. This time it's all right to burn all your bridges. (You can throw away your fat clothes; you'll never need them again if you follow this book.) What you're about to embark on is a total metamorphosis—and you'll never do any wistful looking back. Don't worry, it isn't going to hurt; in fact, I can assure you that it will even feel good.

HALF THE SECRET OF STAYING THIN
One of the main secrets of Staying Thin is really very simple: the thoughts you put in your head are far more important than the food you put in your mouth.

That's why so much of the dieting you tried in

the past only worked for you temporarily. Whether or not the diets were permanently effective had little to do with the chemical or caloric composition of the food you were allowed. Because it wasn't the cheesecake you ultimately devoured that did you in, or the pizza, or even the chocolate cake you so eagerly demolished. It was the things you were *thinking* of that first led you to the forbidden cheesecake, the chocolate, or whatever your Waterloo was. It was your thoughts, and your reaction to those thoughts, that weren't working right for you, not the food itself although it's food you've always blamed.

How can the wrong thoughts make you overeat? Well, let's take hunger and craving, which are two very different needs. Once you respond correctly to them, you've taken a long step toward Staying Thin.

Hunger is the legitimate need of the body for physical nourishment. Craving is an emotional need—a deep, unsatisfiable gnawing feeling. When you respond to craving, you consume food that your body doesn't need, and your waistline shouldn't have. So it's the craving—not the real hunger—that you've got to learn to fight.

Thus, if you're frequently experiencing cravings (rather than hunger), and you're responding to that, then the wrong feeling (craving) is leading you to the wrong response (eating). You'll first have to learn to distinguish between the two, and then learn to substitute other thoughts and actions whenever craving arises.

Therefore, an important part of the secret of

Staying Thin is getting rid of the wrong thoughts and reactions, and putting the right thoughts and responses in your head in the first place. It's those wrong ones that lead to overeating—that mindless, needless pigging-out that has nothing to do with real hunger or the body's real need for nourishment. You'll learn what these wrong thoughts are as you read on, and how to distinguish between them and the positive ones, the ones that tell you it really is time for a light lunch, a balanced dinner, or a sensible snack.

But in order to understand why those cravings crop up, you'll first have to understand why you unconsciously chose to be fat, and why deep down you were comfortable (as well as miserable) with your decision to be overweight. Otherwise, you just aren't going to give up those old wrong patterns.

Remember this: the food didn't just jump off your plate and into your mouth. Something had to go through your mind first that made you want to open your mouth. You may not have been consciously aware of those thoughts, but that's part of what Staying Thin is all about: being aware of what you are thinking, and letting only the constructive thoughts guide your behavior.

Maybe you think I'm placing too much emphasis on something as ephemeral and elusive as the thoughts that flit in and out of our heads. Think again. Think of how powerful your thoughts really are, and how much effect they can have on your body—in more ways than leading you to open a refrigerator door.

For example, we are just beginning to realize how substantially our thoughts and emotions can affect our physical ailments, as well as how much they can help to cure them. Every doctor—and mother—knows how well a sugar pill, a Band-Aid strategically applied, or even some soft words of assurance can work.

Incredible as it seems, some physicians now believe that as many as 75 percent of our ailments are psychosomatic in origin. (If true, that means in effect that three-quarters of the illnesses experienced by our bodies are the result of what is going on in our minds.)

The incredible power of thought that this suggests is supported by cases of people who have undergone experiences that should have caused them intense pain—and yet they didn't feel a thing. Many instances have been reported in medical literature of people who have undergone surgery without anaesthesia, hypnosis, or any external supports, and yet claimed afterwards that they honestly hadn't suffered any pain. In many cases, that's because the thoughts they placed in their heads were able to block the excruciating pain in their bodies.

On a simpler level, we've all had the experience of feeling better when we get to the doctor's office—which is usually just a question of mind over matter. But thoughts can even lead people to believe they underwent an intense and painful operation when no such thing occurred. This has been proven with some fascinating experiments with "sham operations."

In these cases, patients were anaesthetized, scratched up a bit while unconscious, and later told that they had been operated on with total success. And to hear these patients tell it, they genuinely were successful, too. Because whatever pain or discomfort the patients had experienced before was eliminated or substantially reduced by the sham operations.

Now, if thoughts can keep people from feeling intense pain, can cause their bodies to start malfunctioning, and can lead them to believe they had an operation they never had, don't you think thoughts can keep you from performing a simple little act like putting a piece of chocolate cake to your lips?

Perhaps you're beginning to understand why the "diet" presented in this book doesn't consist of a regimen of monotonous foods. You can eat whatever you choose to have (or whatever your doctor tells you to eat or not eat). What you really have to work on now is changing the way you think and how you respond to those thoughts. That's part of the secret of Staying Thin.

But the Stay Thin program also consists of another change that you must make, because there's more to your life than just the thoughts which pop in and out of your head. Obviously you do not live in a vacuum: you talk to friends; you go places; you pass restaurants; you watch television (and commercials); you read newspapers, magazines and books; maybe you even have one of those teen-age sons who comes in from the baseball game, and eats a quarter of a pound of cookies, a bag of potato chips, and a pizza (in that order) in front of you.

And you know, and I know, that there's one thing that keeps popping out at you in this world with equinoctial regularity: **Food.**

From the time we are young, we learn that it's good to cultivate will power and control. But that doesn't mean we have to spend all of our later years challenging it unnecessarily. There's nothing virtuous (or constructive) about placing a plate of freshly baked brownies in front of a new dieter and saying "resist." Likewise, it's better to have cupboards which are *not* filled with illicit temptations than to have a kitchen filled with impossible-to-resist goodies. The job of Staying Thin should be made as easy as possible. And as graceful.

Therefore, the other aspect of this program consists of making changes in your external environment and in the actual way that you approach eating. The purpose of these changes is to help you handle the problem of living in a world where food is always around you, everywhere you look. Because it is often cues from the external environment that make the wrong thoughts pop into your head, if you limit the cues you've at least got a fighting chance.

Now, maybe you think that making some minor changes in your habits and environment requires more stick-to-it-iveness than you have. In the past, you've become unglued when you tried to change your ways, and rapidly reverted to the old habits after a day or two.

Yes, it does require some discipline and self control, but you do have it in you. Almost all of you have, at various times, tried the Diet of the Day: the Scarsdale, the Stillman, the Atkins, mine, etc. All of these required a lot of self-control: you *could* have this on certain days; you *couldn't* have that on others, and so on. If you had the will power to stick to those for a while, you certainly have the will power to make, and stick to, a few basic rules about your own day-to-day eating patterns. Rules, by the way, which are a lot easier to adhere to than a diet, and require far less sacrifice on your part.

And now down to basics.

HOW IT ALL STARTED

The Stay Thin method is based on a popular and successful psychological technique called behavior modification. The purpose of this technique is to help you control your eating habits by changing the behavior—not the causes of it—that made you a problem eater in the first place.

Years ago, psychologists posited the notion that a majority of our problems stemmed from the first few years of our lives. The way to cure these problems, they believed, was to dredge up the traumas and memories of those earlier years and then work them through.

Dr. David Wolpe, a professor of psychiatry at Temple University's School of Medicine, thought otherwise. He didn't deny that many of our problems could be traced back to our earliest years, but his research showed that patients didn't have to spend all those hours (and dollars!) dealing with those childhood traumas again in order to be cured. He found that unpleasant feelings and unproductive behavior could be changed simply by altering our thoughts and actions in the *present*.

Over the years, behavioral techniques have been developed to help people change undesirable behavior, curb irrational (or inexpedient) reactions like phobias, excessive timidity (or aggression), and nervous habits. They have also been found to work especially well for weight loss and maintenance.

These techniques, when used for weight control, demand specific changes in day-to-day living: you will learn to break the chain of your bad habits, and to substitute positive new patterns for those old self-destructive ones. You'll learn a new way of reacting not only to food, but more importantly, to the stress that leads to overeating. In short, you will learn to be aware of and then control your eating behavior.

More and more doctors, particularly psychiatrists and therapists who specialize in handling obesity disorders, are finding that behavior modification is the best—some say the only—way to handle the problem of keeping your weight down once you've lost it in the first place.

That's not to say that conventional psychotherapy, hypnosis, and other techniques don't work for weight loss. They do. But they generally have only a limited success because they rarely attack and change the basic behavioral formula that leads most people to become overweight in the first place, namely that (psychological) Stress leads to a (physical) response which is inappropriate: overeating.

The main advantage of conventional therapy for the compulsive overeater is that it may help reduce the overall amount of stress in that person's life. With less stress, there's less tendency to overeat. But usually, the results are not dramatic. And as everyone knows, the process of therapy is time-consuming and expensive. Moreover, it requires that the patient find a therapist with whom he or she can comfortably work, preferably one who is knowledgeable about the unique problems of overweight people.

Behavior modification can be done on your own. *You,* in effect can be your own therapist. And the basic principles can be learned by reading a book.

You are holding the book—and the solution to your problems—in your hands.

No, I'm not saying that it's enough just to read this book and *voilà,* you'll Stay Thin forever. Reading *any* book without doing anything about it is never enough to effect a complete behavioral overhaul. (If that were true, we could all read the Bible and be perfectly good.) You have to apply what you read to your own life. You have to be prepared to do some work to change your thoughts, your environment, and your eating patterns. And if that seems too strenuous for you, just think of how much effort you put into eating!

What this book can do for you is to make you *aware* of your present behavior, show you what's wrong with it, and point out the ways—the practical methods—by which you can change it. You'll read case histories of people—mostly patients of mine—who have had the same kinds of problems you have had, and who have conquered them.

You'll see that, fortunately, the changes you must make in your thinking and behavior are simple. And it's been proven time and time again, with hundreds of my patients and thousands of others who have used behavior modification to Stay Thin, that these principles work.

And they can work for *you*.

HOW THE STAY THIN
METHOD WAS DEVELOPED
I know the Stay Thin method works because it has been used successfully by so many of my patients, who, prior to trying this technique, had rapidly lost weight, and then just as quickly put it back on again. The Stay Thin method spelled salvation for them and finally ended the yo-yo syndrome which many had despaired was their destiny.

The method did not evolve overnight. A few years ago, I helped develop one of the fastest methods ever devised for losing weight: the protein-sparing modified fast. Patients who went on this type of diet (under strict medical supervision) were able to lose approximately a pound a day for the first month, and then three to five pounds a week for as long as they remained on the regimen.

But the fact that weight loss occurred so rapidly with this method created an unusual situation. My patients quickly reached the weight desired, enjoyed their new slim reflections in the mirror for a while, but then some began to climb right back up there again afterward. It was almost as if they hadn't wanted to stay thin. Few had adjusted their heads (and their environment) to their new bodies.

Naturally, it was satisfying to find myself with an office full of thin patients—an uncommon situation for a bariatric physician. But when I talked with the patients about their weight loss, I soon realized that many had serious problems.

Most of them had convinced themselves earlier that weight was their major obstacle in life, and that if they could overcome that problem, all of their other difficulties would miraculously and instantaneously vanish. Instead, things were often worse, because without a weight problem, they had to face their *real* problems in life—without any experience in dealing with them directly or more importantly, without any excuses.

Linda, for example, was only thirty-six, but she had already developed a triple chin. When she realized that her husband had lost all interest in her, and was sneaking out at nights to see his bookkeeper, she decided to make a concerted effort and succeeded in losing sixty-two pounds in three months.

Fine. But afterwards, when she was down to only one chin, she discovered that her husband was *still* seeing his bookkeeper. She then had to face the realization that her weight loss made no difference to him. He simply was no longer interested in *her*—fat *or* thin. Once she couldn't use the excuse of her fatness to rationalize his lack of desire toward her and realized that her weight was not the cause of her marital problems, or the solution to them, she marched right back to the refrigerator again. What the hell?

Jill turned to eating to give her something to do. She had always been big-boned, it's true. But she didn't have a real weight problem until her three children all graduated from high school and left home. Then, she felt that nobody really needed her anymore, and that there was nothing for her to do at home during the day—but nibble. It didn't take long for her to graduate into half-sizes, D cups, and baggy house dresses.

Jill decided that if she lost weight, she could do some volunteer work, brush up her old tennis again, and meet with her friends more often. But she was lazy, and even after losing thirty-five pounds, she still sat around the house all day. Reaching her goal weight didn't make the clock move any faster in the lonely afternoons. Furthermore, at home alone, her weight loss went unnoticed, and soon she was nibbling—and overweight—again.

And Jack V. admits that he was "born with a chocolate spoon in [his] mouth." As a result of his childhood chubbiness, which developed into teenage tubbiness, "I couldn't make it socially," he ruefully recalls. "I was known as a fatty, and wasn't in the right crowd at school. I felt that the other kids were talking about me—and they probably were. I was always uncomfortable socially. I became so used to rejection by others, that after a while, I didn't even bother to compete. I said what the heck, withdrew to a stamp collection, and let myself get even fatter."

At the age of twenty-four, when he was not only a virgin but had never even gone out on a date, he dramatically lost eighty-five pounds. Since he no longer had the I'm-so-fat-she'll-turn-me-down excuse, he finally got up the courage to ask a girl to the movies. But, as bad luck would have it, she turned him down. Devastated, and petrified because he no longer had his weight as an excuse for being rejected, in just one month he put back forty of those lost pounds.

Listening to these patients' problems, and other similar ones, I came to understand why there are so many failed dieters in America today. We give people diets that work, but then we drive them right back to self-destructive overeating because we don't do anything to help them maintain their proper weight afterwards. Furthermore, we instill in them the unrealistic notion that being thin is the shortcut to everything they want in life, and neglect the fact that being thin solves no problems but the weight problem.

Once they are thin, ex-fatties still face the same emotional and external problems they had when they were overweight: in fact, those problems may be more overwhelming to them than ever. First, they no longer have an excuse for the problem. And secondly, they still know only one way to handle the stresses that contributed to those problems in the first place—overeating. We weren't teaching people how not to take up the old patterns when confronted with the tensions and strains of their lives. We weren't teaching them new methods to deal with stress.

Let's face it. All diets come down to pretty much the same thing, no matter how "revolutionary" they claim to be: consume fewer calories (and, in some cases, expend more energy by exercising). But staying thin is another—and often harder—matter. I became aware of this as I saw more and more of my patients easily conquering their weight problems only to find themselves at a loss as to how to stay that way while trying to straighten out the rest of their muddled lives.

The answer to their problems turned out to be the formal and informal Stay Thin programs we established in my offices. This book is a modification of what patients in my classes have learned, an expansion of work being done by a number of doctors and psychologists in this field (including what I've been able to contribute as a bariatric physician), plus the research and work of the staff behavioral psychologists who actually teach these Stay Thin courses.

When the program was tested, we found that people who had yo-yoed even over a dozen times, were finally able to keep their weight at a desirable level (some for over two years now) as a result of the Stay Thin techniques.

In this book I've included many case histories of patients in the classes, problems they encountered and solutions that worked for them. No doubt you'll be able to identify with these people, since they've gone through what you too have experienced. But if your situation and problems are *so* unique that you don't find yourself in any of their stories, reading about others should still help you raise your consciousness, so that you can ultimately liberate yourself from the tyranny of your compulsion to overeat.

Patients who faithfully followed the Stay Thin method found that for the first time in their long dieting life they were finally able to do the two things you must do if you're finally going to Stay Thin: *Be Aware* and *be in control*.

In order to keep your weight off, you must learn to buy, order, and consume food *consciously*—at every step of the way. For example, your hand must no longer dart out to the peanut dish without your really realizing it, just because the conversation is hitting a snag. You must become superaware of your home, your office, your dining out, and your whole eating environment: the pitfalls, the treacherous spots, and the temptations.

Then, with this increased awareness, you'll learn to control all these situations. And the end result will be that you will *consciously choose* exactly which foods to put into your mouth, along with when and how much. You will at last be in complete control of you environment and eating activities—and not the other way around.

For most yo-yos, or recidivists, it's tough to walk into a supermarket, a restaurant, a wedding buffet, or a skinny friend's ample kitchen. But by the time you finish this book, you should be able to handle all those situations, and many more, without feeling deprived—or depressed.

Although it's easier, and sometimes more pleasant, to learn by participating in a group program, it's not necessary for you to join a class or a doctor's group in order to undertake the Stay Thin method. You can do it now, on your own.

In fact, by reading this far, you've already started.

As we continue, I will pinpoint the pitfalls and temptations you will encounter and show you how to control them by being aware of each and the actions it may precipitate. From your own pantry shelf to the lavish office Christmas party or the sumptuous Sunday brunch, you'll learn to decide, for yourself, what you'll eat. And, as a result, the new you will be your own creation, not merely a production of some diet expert.

3
Eating
and Exercising
the Stay Thin Way

The focus of this book is on changing your thoughts, increasing your motivation, and altering your environment (or helping you cope with it) so that you will be able to Stay Thin. But no matter how much you change your thinking, or the concrete world around you, you aren't going to be able to accomplish very much if you laze around the house all day, and, to put it bluntly, eat like a pig.

Indeed, basics like proper eating and exercising are often forgotten by people when they first enter our Stay Thin program or read a book such as this. That's because they think that attending classes, or reading a book, will do everything for them, and that they no longer have to do anything for themselves.

That's why I'm going to backtrack a bit before we get to the heart of this program, and devote this early chapter to two basics that must be followed while you read this book, and for that matter, all through your life: Proper eating and proper exercising.

PROPER EATING

In order to choose the right foods, and the proper diet for you, you should understand what makes you fat. Put as simply as possible—fat is just stored energy. Your body needs a certain amount of energy to function each day. Exactly how much energy depends upon how active you are. And if you take in more energy than your body can use, the excess is stored as fat.

It's that simple: ingest more calories than you expend and they have to turn to fat. If you cut down on the amount of food you eat, the body is forced to use its own fat for energy and you lose weight. (The utilization of about 3,500 extra calories equals the loss of one pound.) But if you burn about the same number of calories as you take in, you can maintain your weight forever.

Thus, the first thing you must do is to figure out how many calories a day will allow you to maintain your ideal weight. But in order to really do this properly, you should establish your activity level: low, medium or high.

Now, you low-activity people know who you are. You most likely have a sedentary job, you probably like to sit and watch television or take it easy in the evenings, you prefer taking a car, bus, or taxi to using your legs, and, if you bother to exercise at all, it's such a minimal amount that it could accomplish no more than alleviating some of your guilt about how badly you're caring for your body.

If, however, you exercise a few times a week, make it a point to walk whenever possible, and engage in some sport at least once a week, you most likely fall into the mid-range. And, unfortunately, only the few of you who run or jog every day, work out frequently, and seek out physical activity instead of wallowing in indolence, fit into the high activity level.

Now, to establish how many calories you may have each day, look at the following chart and locate your weight on the left hand side of the page. Then, choose your level of activity (low, mid, or high range). Next, come down the list of numbers for that level until you reach the one that is parallel to your weight. That's the number of calories you need. For example, if your weight is 125, and you are moderately active, you can maintain this weight if you ingest 1,500 calories a day.

CALORIC INTAKE TO MAINTAIN WEIGHT

WEIGHT (pounds)	LOW ACTIVITY (calories)	MID RANGE (calories)	HIGH ACTIVITY (calories)
100	1,000	1,200	1,400
105	1,050	1,260	1,470
110	1,100	1,320	1,540
115	1,150	1,380	1,610
120	1,200	1,440	1,680

WEIGHT (pounds)	LOW ACTIVITY (calories)	MID RANGE (calories)	HIGH ACTIVITY (calories)
125	1,250	1,500	1,750
130	1,300	1,560	1,820
135	1,350	1,620	1,890
140	1,400	1,680	1,960
145	1,450	1,740	2,030
150	1,500	1,800	2,100
155	1,550	1,860	2,170
160	1,600	1,920	2,240
165	1,650	1,980	2,310
170	1,700	2,040	2,380
175	1,750	2,100	2,450
180	1,800	2,160	2,520
185	1,850	2,220	2,590
190	1,900	2,280	2,660
195	1,950	2,340	2,730
200	2,000	2,400	2,800
205	2,050	2,460	2,870
210	2,100	2,520	2,940
215	2,150	2,580	3,010
220	2,200	2,640	3,080
225	2,250	2,700	3,150

If you *really* want to understand calories, and what you can eat, buy a comprehensive calorie dictionary. But don't bother with those little pocket or paperback ones. In those, the foods you want to eat usually won't be listed, or they'll be listed in the wrong amounts and you'll end up guessing at their caloric values, and invariably underestimating them, i.e., cheating.

The best type of calorie dictionary is one that

specifically lists food items by brand name since there's surprising variation among the same type of product. For example, say you have an overpowering urge for a chocolate chip cookie tonight. Obviously, you shouldn't give in to it. But if you do, you'll see from a brand-name calorie dictionary that you're better off with a Nabisco Snap at twenty-one calories than with a Keebler Old-Fashioned Chocolate Chip cookie at eighty.

In fact, even among diet goods there's a lot of variation among brands. For instance, one tablespoon of Wish-Bone Low Calorie French dressing is twenty-three calories, while one tablespoon of the same by Tillie Lewis is only three. Since you'll probably use more than one tablespoon of dressing on a salad, the difference can add up.

Indeed, even among foods with negligible calorie counts, there's some variation among brands. A cube of Herb-Ox bouillon is six calories, while a cube of Wylers (with no salt added) is eleven. Sure, that's only five calories. But if you drink five cups of bouillon a day to curb your appetite, saving twenty-five calories would allow you an extra half a small orange in your meal plan for that day.

If you want to devise your own meal plan, make a list of those things you really like, should have, or can eat. Then, check their calorie content in your dictionary and establish a diet for yourself that stays within the daily calorie range you determined earlier.

Or if you prefer you can use one that I often give my patients because it's less restricted than most diets. If you follow this plan, do not circle more than three-four items for breakfast, five items for lunch, and a maximum of seven items for dinner.

Be sure you take into account while planning your meals that the single most important factor for insuring dietary adequacy is the variability of food selection. The diets supplied here are varied and will supply reasonable amounts of the vitamins and minerals needed for normal functioning, but I do recommend vitamin-mineral supplementation for the following reasons:

1. There is a tremendous amount of individual variation when it comes to the way in which individuals absorb and utilize vitamins. It is quite impossible for a nutritionist to say whether an individual does or does not need a specific vitamin supplement unless an extensive dietary history along with certain biochemical tests are done on the person's blood and urine.

2. The nutrient content of the same food raised or grown in different areas can vary enormously and it is therefore impossible to know what we are getting on a day-to-day basis.

3. There is a significant loss of vitamins (especially the Bs and C) through storage and preparation of foods. To minimize these losses, foods should not be overcooked, and fresh produce should be used whenever possible.

I would advise you to purchase a good vitamin-mineral supplement at your drug store or reliable health food store. Also, take the supplement *after* meals to minimize the risk of stomach upset (some people are sensitive to vitamin B1). Skipping a day now and then presents no problem since four to five supplements a week will be quite adequate.

PROPER EXERCISING

The next thing you must start when reading this book—and continue for the rest of your life—is a good exercise program. You may already have your own favorite exercises, which probably means that there are some exercises you hate to do less than others. But if you do not have one, you can do the ten exercises below that I frequently suggest for my patients, since each one firms up different parts of your body.

In order to establish a lifetime exercise program, you should build up to it slowly. The best way to do that is to steadily increase the number of the exercises you do each week until you reach your optimal level (that should take about a month). In addition, before starting your actual exercises each day, you should run through the following three warm-up exercises to get you ready. (If you already jog or run daily, you can skip jogging in place and jumping rope.)

WARM-UP 1—STRETCHING Stand with your legs apart, your knees bent, and your arms at your sides. Tighten your buttocks. Then, reach for the ceiling with your right arm while your left one remains in place.

Then, reach up with your left arm while dropping the right one back to your side.

Start at five for the first week and build up to twenty by the end of the month.

WARM-UP 2—JOGGING IN PLACE Stand with your feet together and jog in place for a couple of minutes.

WARM-UP 3—JUMPING ROPE Just jump as if you were jumping rope. (Naturally, if you have a jump rope, use it.)

Start at eleven jumps and work up to twenty by the end of the month.

EXERCISE 1—FOR THE BUTTOCKS, THIGHS, HIPS AND CALVES Get on your hands and knees and raise your knee till it forms a straight line with your shoulder. Kick straight back and also to the side as far as you can. Alternate legs.

Start at ten and add five a week until you reach twenty-five.

EXERCISE 2—FOR THE BUTTOCKS, HIPS, CALVES, AND THIGHS Lie on your back with your feet together and your knees bent toward you. Tighten your stomach muscles and bring your knees to your chest. Then, keeping your legs off the floor, stretch them out as far as you can.

Start at ten and add five a week until you reach twenty-five.

EXERCISE 3—FOR THE BUTTOCKS Lie on your stomach and put your hands under your pelvis. Lift your knees up toward your head. Tighten your buttocks muscles and slap your thighs together.

Start at ten and add five a week until you reach twenty-five.

Summary of essential nutrients

Essential nutrients	Function in the body	Good food sources	Comments
Protein	Required for growth, maintenance, and repair of body tissues. Helps to make hemoglobin, form antibodies to fight infection, and supply energy.	Meat, poultry, fish, eggs, milk, cheese, soybeans, beans, peas, grains, and nuts.	Foods of animal origin contain protein of better nutritional value than foods of plant origin.
Carbohydrates (starches, sugars, and celluloses)	Starches and sugars are major sources of energy for internal and external work and to maintain body temperature. Celluloses furnish bulk in diet.	Grains (wheat, oats, corn, rice) and grain products (flour, bread, cereal, macaroni, etc.), sugar, jams and jellies, candy, soft drinks, honey, and most fruits and vegetables.	Excess carbohydrates in diet are converted into fat and are stored in the body.
Fats	Concentrated source of energy. Carry fat-soluble vitamins and help body to use them. Fats also make up part of cell structure, cushion vital organs; some contain linoleic acid, believed to be essential for health.	Butter, margarine, cooking and salad oils, cream, most cheeses, nuts, bacon, fatty meats, and—to some extent—whole milk, eggs, chocolate, and most meat.	"Unsaturated" fat or linoleic acid found in most vegetable oils; poultry and fish oils have more than animal fats.
Minerals: Calcium	Builds bones and teeth; aids in proper functioning of muscles, heart, and nerves; helps in blood coagulation.	Milk, hard cheese, and in kale, mustard, turnip and collard greens. Also some in oysters, shrimp, salmon, clams, and in other dairy products.	Calcium is the most abundant mineral in the body.

Summary of essential nutrients (continued)

Essential nutrients	Function in the body	Good food sources	Comments
Iron	One of the constituents of hemoglobin, which carries oxygen to the tissues by blood circulation. Iron is present in all body cells.	All kinds of liver are the best source of iron; also: meat, egg yolk, legumes, molasses, dark green leafy vegetables, peaches, prunes, apricots, raisins, and food made with enriched flour or cereal.	Iron deficiency is most common in growing children, adolescent girls, pregnant or nursing women.
Phosphorus	Builds bones and teeth (with other minerals); important in a number of body systems involving fats, carbohydrates, salts, and enzymes.	Milk, cheese, egg yolk, meat, fish, fowl, legumes, nuts, whole-grain cereals.	Some forms of phosphorus are not utilized if the vitamin D level is inadequate in the diet.
Iodine	Required to regulate the exchange of food for energy.	Iodized salt best protection; also salt water fish.	The need for iodine is increased in adolescence and during pregnancy.
Potassium	Needed to maintain fluid balance within the cell; regulates muscular and nervous irritability; necessary for regular heart rhythm.	Meat, fish, fowl, cereals, fruits, vegetables.	Deficiency in diet is uncommon, but may occur in connection with some diseases.

44

Sodium	Protects body against excessive fluid loss, regulates muscle and nerve irritability, and maintains water balance.	Table salt, meat, fish, fowl, milk, eggs, and sodium compounds	Excessive salt intake dangerous for persons subject to hypertension and kidney disorders.
Fluorine	In small quantities protects the teeth against cavities. In larger quantities, fluorine causes mottling of the teeth.	Milk, eggs, and fish; many communities add low concentrations of fluorine to drinking water.	Prolonged high intake of fluorine may cause skeletal abnormalities.
Other minerals which are considered essential for good health are: chlorine, sulfur, magnesium, manganese, copper, zinc, cobalt, and molybdenum. In most cases, diet provides adequate intake.			
Vitamin A	Important for skeletal growth and normal tooth structure; necessary for healthy mucous membranes in mouth, nose, throat, digestive and urinary tracts; and essential for night vision.	Fish-liver oils, liver, butter, cream, milk, cheese, egg yolk, dark green and yellow vegetables, yellow fruits, and fortified margarine.	Fat soluble; destroyed by oxidation and very high temperatures.
Vitamin B₁ (Thiamine)	Necessary to help convert sugar and starches into energy.	Pork, liver, heart, kidney, milk, yeast, whole-grain and enriched cereals and breads, soybeans, legumes, peanuts, and wheat germ.	Quickly destroyed by heat in neutral or alkaline solutions.

Summary of essential nutrients (continued)

Essential nutrients	Function in the body	Good food sources	Comments
Vitamin B_2 (Riboflavin)	Essential link in the body's use of protein, carbohydrates, and fats for energy.	Milk, powdered whey, liver, kidney, heart, meats, eggs, green leafy vegetables, dried yeast.	Decomposes quickly in light or in alkaline solutions.
Vitamin B_6 (Pyridoxine, pyridoxal, pyridoxamine)	Important for the body's use of protein, carbohydrates, and fat; aids in formation of hemoglobin.	Wheat germ, meat, liver, kidneys, whole-grain cereals, soybeans, peanuts, corn; some in milk and green vegetables.	Water soluble; destroyed by ultraviolet light and heat.
Vitamin B_{12} (Cobalamin)	Essential for forming red blood cells; helps in forming all cells in body and in functioning of nervous system.	Milk, eggs, cheese, liver, kidney, muscle meats contain small amounts needed for normal body functioning.	Inactivated by air or light; water soluble.
Folic acid	Needed for use of protein in body and for regeneration of blood cells.	Green leafy vegetables, liver, kidney, yeast, and—in lesser quantities—many foods.	Easily inactivated in sunlight and acid solutions.
Pantothenic acid	Necessary for the body's use of carbohydrates, fats, and protein in conjunction with other substances.	Almost universally present in plant and animal tissue. Loss of 50% in milling of flour; 33% lost in cooking meat.	Water soluble; destroyed easily by dry heat and alkaline.

46

Vitamin	Function	Sources	Properties
Niacin	Active in normal functioning of tissues, particularly of the skin, gastrointestinal tract, and nervous system; with other vitamins, used in converting carbohydrates to energy.	Lean meat, liver, kidney, whole-grain and enriched cereals and breads, green vegetables, peanuts, yeast.	Water soluble, stable to heat, air, light.
Biotin	Essential for the functioning of many body systems and use of food for energy.	Liver, kidney, molasses, milk, yeast, egg yolk, and green vegetables.	Water soluble; quite stable in heat, air, and light.
Vitamin C (Ascorbic acid)	Essential for the formation of collagen, a protein which supports the body structures; needed for the absorption of iron, some proteins, and folic acid.	Citrus fruits, strawberries, cantaloupe, tomatoes, cabbage, potatoes, green peppers, and broccoli.	Water soluble; destroyed by heat, air, and light, as well as by aging, drying, and copper contact.
Vitamin D	Promotes normal bone and tooth development; necessary for absorption and stabilization of calcium and phosphorus.	Fish-liver oils, fortified milk, exposure to sunlight; very small amounts in butter, liver, and egg yolks.	Fat soluble; stable to heat and air.
Vitamin E (Tocopherol)	Protects the body's store of vitamin A and the tissue fat from destructive oxidation; also prevents breakdown of red blood corpuscles.	Oils of wheat germ, rice germ, cottonseed, and the germs of other seeds; green leafy vegetables, nuts, and legumes.	Fat soluble; breaks down in presence of lead and iron salts, alkalis, and ultraviolet light.

Summary of essential nutrients (continued)

Essential nutrients	Function in the body	Good food sources	Comments
Vitamin K	Essential for blood clotting.	Green leafy vegetables such as alfalfa, spinach, cabbage; liver.	Fat soluble; unstable to light.
Water	Essential for life; is the solvent for all products of digestion, the medium of body fluids; regulates body temperature.	Beverages, many solid foods (for example, potatoes contain 78% water).	One-half to two-thirds of the body is made up of water.

Courtesy of the American Osteopathic Association

Breakfast—Menu of day

	CALORIES
__ 1½ T. raisins	40
__ ½ c. oatmeal	65
__ ½ c. skim milk	45
	Total 150

__ cereal_____

Dairy, Eggs

__ 2, 3 eggs whites + margarine	50,70
__ 4, 6 egg whites + margarine	90,140
__ 4 oz., 8 oz. skim milk	45,90
__ ¼ c., ½ c. cottage cheese	50,100

Fresh Fruit

__ ½ grapefruit	50
__ ½ orange, ½ apple	40,40
__ ½ banana	45
__ _____	
__ ½ c. canned peaches	40
__ ½ c. canned pineapple	50

Total (Breakfast)   C

Lunch—Menu of day

__ 3 oz. boiled shrimp	100
__ 1 oz. cocktail sauce	15
__ ½ fresh orange	40
	Total 155

Dairy, Meat

__ 1 oz., 2 oz. beef	60,120
__ ¼ c., ½ c. cottage cheese	60,100
__ 4 oz., 8 oz. plain yogurt	75,150
__ 1½ oz., 3 oz. tuna fish	50,100

Vegetables

__ 6 oz., 12 oz. vegetable soup	30,60
__ 1 slice tomato, lettuce wedge	10,10
__ 6 oz., 12 oz. tossed salad	10,20

Fresh Fruit

__ ½ grapefruit	50
__ ½ orange, ½ apple	40,40
__ ½ banana	45
__	
__ ½ c. canned peaches	40
__ ½ c. canned pineapple	50

Miscellaneous

__ 1 oz. diet dressing	30
__ 1 oz. diet catsup	15
__ 1 tsp. oil, 1 tsp. margarine	40,35
__ ½ bread slice	35

Total (Lunch)   C

Dinner—Menu of day

__ 6 oz. baked chicken	300
__ 2 oz. curry sauce	25
__ 2 broccoli spears	20
__ small tossed salad w/2 tomato wedges	30
__ 1 oz. diet dressing	30
Total	405

Meat

__ 5 oz. turbot	300

Vegetables

__ 2 cucumber sticks	10
__ 1 slice tomato, lettuce wedge	10,10
__ 6 oz., 12 oz. tossed salad	10,20
__ celery or carrot sticks	10,10
__ ½ c. zucchini w/tomato sauce	20
__ 4 apricot halves	50

Fruit

__ ½ grapefruit	50
__ ½ orange, ½ apple	40,40
__ ½ banana	45
__	

__ ½ c. canned peaches	40
__ ½ c. canned pineapple	50

Miscellaneous

__ 1 oz. diet dressing	30
__ 1 oz. diet catsup	15
__ 1 tsp. oil, 1 tsp. margarine	40,35
__ ½ bread slice	35

Total (Dinner)   C

Total (Day)   C

TUESDAY—WEEK 3

Breakfast—Menu of day   CALORIES

__ 3 egg whites	45
__ ¾ tsp. margarine	25
__ ¼ c. cottage cheese	50
__ ¼ melon wedge	30
Total	150

__ cereal

Dairy, Eggs

__ 2, 3 egg whites + margarine	50,70
__ 4, 6 egg whites + margarine	90,140
__ 4 oz., 8 oz. skim milk	45,90
__ ¼ c., ½ c. cottage cheese	50,100

Fresh Fruit

__ ½ grapefruit	50
__ ½ orange, ½ apple	40,40
__ ½ banana	45

__ ½ c. canned peaches	40
__ ½ c. canned pineapple	50

Total (Breakfast)   C

Lunch—Menu of day

__ whole tomato	35
__ ½ c. spring salad	100
__ celery and carrot sticks	10
Total	145

Dairy, Meat

__ 1 oz., 2 oz. beef	60,120
__ ¼ c., ½ c. cottage cheese	50,100
__ 4 oz., 8 oz. plain yogurt	75,150
__ 1½ oz., 3 oz. tuna fish	50,100

Vegetables

__ 6 oz., 12 oz. vegetable soup	30,60
__ 1 slice tomato, lettuce wedge	10,10
__ 6 oz., 12 oz. tossed salad	10,20

Fresh Fruit

__ ½ grapefruit	50
__ ½ orange, ½ apple	40,40
__ ½ banana	45

Miscellaneous

__ 1 oz. diet dressing	30
__ 1 oz. diet catsup	15
__ 1 tsp. oil, 1 tsp. margarine	40,35
__ ½ bread slice	35

Total (Lunch)   C

Dinner—Menu of day

__ 1 c. beef & rice casserole	260
__ 2 oz. tomato sauce	25
__ ½ c. cabbage	15
__ ½ grapefruit	50
__ tossed salad	20
__ 1 oz. diet dressing	30
Total	400

Meat

__ 6 oz. chicken   300

Vegetables

__ 2 cucumber sticks	10
__ 1 slice tomato, lettuce wedge	10,10
__ 6 oz., 12 oz. tossed salad	10,20
__ ½ c. spinach	20
__ ½ c. chilled green bean + onion salad	20

Fruit

__ ½ grapefruit	50
__ ½ orange, ½ apple	40,40
__ ½ banana	45
__ _____	
__ ½ c. canned peaches	40
__ ½ c. canned pineapple	50

Miscellaneous

__ 1 oz. diet dressing	30
__ 1 oz. diet catsup	15
__ 1 tsp. oil, 1 tsp. margarine	40,35
__ ½ bread slice	35

Total (Dinner)   C

Total (Day)   C

WEDNESDAY—WEEK 3

Breakfast—Menu of day   **CALORIES**

__ ½ fresh orange		40
__ 1 fried or poached egg		75
__ 1 tsp. margarine		35
	Total	150

__ cereal _____

Dairy, Eggs

__ 2, 3 egg whites + margarine   50,70

___ 4, 6 egg whites + margarine   90,140
___ 4 oz., 8 oz. skim milk   45,90
___ ¼ c., ½ c. cottage cheese   50,100

Fresh Fruit

___ ½ grapefruit   50
___ ½ orange, ½ apple   40,40
___ ½ banana   45

___ _____

___ ½ c. canned peaches   40
___ ½ c. canned pineapple   50

Total (Breakfast)   C

Lunch—Menu of day

___ Salad Bowl:
    2 oz. turkey   100
    1 slice tomato   10
    shredded lettuce   10
    1 oz. diet dressing   30
                    Total   150

Dairy, Meat

___ 1 oz., 2 oz. beef   60,120
___ ¼ c., ½ c. cottage cheese   50,100
___ 4 oz., 8 oz. plain yogurt   75,150
___ 1½ oz., 3 oz. tuna fish   50,100

Vegetables

___ 6 oz., 12 oz. vegetable soup   30,60
___ 1 slice tomato, lettuce wedge   10,10
___ 6 oz., 12 oz. tossed salad   10,20

Fresh Fruit

___ ½ grapefruit   50
___ ½ orange, ½ apple   40,40
___ ½ banana   45

___ _____

___ ½ c. canned peaches   40
___ ½ c. canned pineapple   50

Miscellaneous

__ 1 oz. diet dressing	30
__ 1 oz. diet catsup	15
__ 1 tsp. oil, 1 tsp. margarine	40,35
__ ½ bread slice	35

Total (Lunch)   C

Dinner—Menu of day

__ Tuna casserole		250
__ ½ c. cauliflower		10
__ ½ c. carrots		20
__ Salad-lettuce wedge, 2 tomato slices		30
__ 1 oz. diet dressing		30
__ ½ melon		60
	Total	400

Vegetables

__ 2 cucumber sticks	10
__ 1 tomato slice, lettuce wedge	10,10
__ 6 oz., 12 oz. tossed salad	10,20
__ celery or carrot sticks	10,10
__ 2 broccoli spears	20
__ ½ c. grated radish, carrot, cabbage salad on lettuce leaf	20

Fruit

__ ½ grapefruit	50
__ ½ orange, ½ apple	40,40
__ ½ banana	45
__	
__ ½ c. canned peaches	40
__ ½ c. canned pineapple	50

Miscellaneous

__ 1 oz. diet dressing	30
__ 1 oz. diet catsup	15
__ 1 tsp. oil, 1 tsp. margarine	40,35
__ ½ bread slice	35

Total (Dinner)   C

Total (Day)   C

THURSDAY—WEEK 3

Breakfast—Menu of day   CALORIES

__ ½ grapefruit	50
__ ¾ c. Special K	60
__ ½ c. skim milk	45
	Total 155

__ cereal_____

Dairy, Eggs

__ 2, 3 egg whites + margarine	50,70
__ 4, 6 egg whites + margarine	90,140
__ 4 oz., 8 oz. skim milk	45,90
__ ¼ c., ½ c. cottage cheese	50,100

Fresh Fruit

__ ½ grapefruit	50
__ ½ orange, ½ apple	40,40
__ ½ banana	45

__ ½ c. canned peaches	40
__ ½ c. canned pineapple	50

Total (Breakfast)   C

Lunch—Menu of day

__ ½ c. carrot salad	45
__ 1 oz. lemon yogurt	25
__ 6 oz. soup	30
__ 1½ oz. tuna	50
	Total 150

Dairy, Meat

__ 1 oz., 2 oz. beef	60,120
__ ¼ c., ½ c. cottage cheese	50,100
__ 4 oz., 8 oz. plain yogurt	75,150
__ 1½ oz., 3 oz. tuna fish	50,100

Vegetables

__ 6 oz., 12 oz. vegetable soup	30,60

___ 1 slice tomato, lettuce wedge   10,10
___ 6 oz., 12 oz. tossed salad   10,20

Fresh Fruit

___ ½ grapefruit   50
___ ½ orange, ½ apple   40,40
___ ½ banana   45
_____
___ ½ c. canned peaches   40
___ ½ c. canned pineapple   50

Miscellaneous

___ 1 oz. diet dressing   30
___ 1 oz. diet catsup   15
___ 1 tsp. oil, 1 tsp. margarine   40,35
___ ½ bread slice   35

Total (Lunch)   C

Dinner—Menu of day

___ 5 oz. sirloin steak   300
___ ½ baked potato   45
___ tossed salad w/slice tomato + onion   25
___ 1 oz. diet dressing   30
                              Total   400

Meat

___ 5 oz. turbot   300

Vegetables

___ 2 cucumber sticks   10
___ 1 tomato slice, lettuce wedge   10,10
___ 6 oz., 12 oz. tossed salad   10,20
___ celery or carrot sticks   10,10
___ broiled tomato half w/Italian dressing   30
_____

Fruit

___ ½ grapefruit   50
___ ½ orange, ½ apple   40,40

57

__ ½ banana	45

__ ½ c. canned peaches	40
__ ½ c. canned pineapple	50

Miscellaneous

__ 1 oz. diet dressing	30
__ 1 oz. diet catsup	15
__ 1 tsp. oil, 1 tsp. margarine	40,35
__ ½ bread slice	35

Total (Dinner)   C

Total (Day)   C

FRIDAY—WEEK 3

Breakfast—Menu of day   **CALORIES**

__ ½ c. Pettijohns		75
__ ½ c. skim milk		45
__ ½ orange		40
	Total	160

__ cereal_____

Dairy, Eggs

__ 2, 3 egg whites + margarine	50,70
__ 4, 6 egg whites + margarine	90,140
__ 4 oz, 8 oz. skim milk	45,90
__ ¼ c., ½ c. cottage cheese	50,100

Fresh Fruit

__ ½ grapefruit	50
__ ½ orange, ½ apple	40,40
__ ½ banana	45

__ ½ c. canned peaches	40
__ ½ c. canned pineapple	50

Total (Breakfast)   C

Lunch—Menu of day

__ 4 oz. beef broth w/onion	10
__ 1 tomato	35
__ ½ c. spring salad	100
Total	145

Dairy, Meat

__ 1 oz., 2 oz. beef	60,120
__ ¼ c., ½ c. cottage cheese	50,100
__ 4 oz., 8 oz. plain yogurt	75,150
__ 1½ oz., 3 oz. tuna fish	50,100

Vegetables

__ 6 oz., 12 oz. vegetable soup	30,60
__ 1 slice tomato, lettuce wedge	10,10
__ 6 oz., 12 oz. tossed salad	10,20

Fresh Fruit

__ ½ grapefruit	50
__ ½ orange, ½ apple	40,40
__ ½ banana	45

__ ½ c. canned peaches	40
__ ½ c. canned pineapple	50

Miscellaneous

__ 1 oz. diet dressing	30
__ 1 oz. diet catsup	15
__ 1 tsp. oil, 1 tsp. margarine	40,35
__ ½ bread slice	35

Total (Lunch)	C

Dinner—Menu of day

__ 5 oz. baked turbot	300
__ ½ c. stewed tomatoes	20
__ lettuce wedge	10
__ 1 oz. diet dressing	30
__ ½ baked apple	40
Total	400

Meat

__ 6 oz. chicken	300

Vegetables

__ 2 cucumber sticks	10
__ 1 tomato slice, lettuce wedge	10,10
__ 6 oz., 12 oz. tossed salad	10,20
__ celery or carrot sticks	10,10
__ ½ c. beet & onion salad	30
__ ½ c. spinach	20

Fruit

__ ½ grapefruit	50
__ ½ orange, ½ apple	40,40
__ ½ banana	45
__ _____	
__ ½ c. canned peaches	40
__ ½ c. canned pineapple	50

Miscellaneous

__ 1 oz. diet dressing	30
__ 1 oz. diet catsup	15
__ 1 tsp. oil, 1 tsp. margarine	40,35
__ ½ bread slice	35

Total (Dinner)	C
Total (Day)	C

SATURDAY—WEEK 3

Breakfast—Menu of day	CALORIES
__ ½ c. drained peaches	40
__ 1 c. puffed rice	55
__ ½ c. skim milk	45
Total	140
__ cereal _____	

Dairy, Eggs

__ 2, 3 egg whites + margarine	50,70
__ 4, 6 egg whites + margarine	90,140
__ 4 oz., 8 oz. skim milk	45,90
__ ¼ c., ½ c. cottage cheese	50,100

Fresh Fruit

__ ½ grapefruit	50
__ ½ orange, ½ apple	40,40
__ ½ banana	45
_____	
__ ½ c. canned peaches	40
__ ½ c. canned pineapple	50

Total (Breakfast)   C

Lunch—Menu of day

Salad Bowl:

__ 3 oz. salmon		120
__ 1 T. chopped onion		5
__ 1 tomato wedge		10
__ shredded lettuce		10
	Total	145

Dairy, Meat

__ 1 oz., 2 oz. beef	60,120
__ ¼ c., ½ c. cottage cheese	50,100
__ 4 oz., 8 oz. plain yogurt	75,150
__ 1½ oz., 3 oz. tuna fish	50,100

Vegetables

__ 6 oz., 12 oz. vegetable soup	30,60
__ 1 slice tomato, lettuce wedge	10,10
__ 6 oz., 12 oz. tossed salad	20,20

Fresh Fruit

__ ½ grapefruit	50
__ ½ orange, ½ apple	40,40
__ ½ banana	45
_____	
__ ½ c. canned peaches	40

__ ½ c. canned pineapple   50

Miscellaneous

__ 1 oz. diet dressing   30
__ 1 oz. diet catsup   15
__ 1 tsp. oil, 1 tsp. margarine   40,35
__ ½ bread slice   35

Total (Lunch)   C

Dinner—Menu of day

__ 4½ oz. turkey   25
__ 2 oz. diet gravy   25
__ ½ baked potato   45
__ 4 brussels sprouts   20
__ Diced apple mold   30
__ 2 slices tomato   20
__ 1 oz. diet dressing   30
                               Total   395

Meat

__ 4 oz. turbot   240

Vegetables

__ 2 cucumber sticks   10
__ 1 slice tomato, lettuce wedge   10,10
__ 6 oz., 12 oz. tossed salad   10,20
__ celery or carrot sticks   10,10
__ ½ c. stewed tomatoes   20

__ _____

Fresh Fruit

__ ½ grapefruit   50
__ ½ orange, ½ apple   40,40
__ ½ banana   45

__ _____

__ ½ c. canned peaches   40
__ ½ c. canned pineapple   50

Miscellaneous

__ 1 oz. diet dressing   30

__ 1 oz. diet catsup	15
__ 1 tsp. oil, 1 tsp. margarine	40,35
__ ½ bread slice	35

Total (Dinner)   C

Total (Day)   C

SUNDAY—WEEK 3

Breakfast—Menu of Day   CALORIES

__ ¾ c. cornflakes	80
__ ½ c. skim milk	45
__ ¼ c. peaches	20
	Total 145

__ cereal _____

Dairy, Eggs

__ 2, 3 egg whites + margarine	50,70
__ 4, 6 egg whites + margarine	90,140
__ 4 oz., 8 oz. skim milk	45,90
__ ¼ c., ½ c. cottage cheese	50,100

Fresh Fruit

__ ½ grapefruit	50
__ ½ orange, ½ apple	40,40
__ ½ banana	45
__ _____	
__ ½ c. canned peaches	40
__ ½ c. canned pineapple	50

Total (Breakfast)   C

Lunch—Menu of day

__ 4 oz. plain yogurt	75
__ ½ c. blueberries	45
__ 6 oz. vegetable soup	30
	Total 145

Dairy, Meat

__ 1 oz., 2 oz. beef	60,120
__ ¼ c., ½ c. cottage cheese	50,100
__ 4 oz., 8 oz. plain yogurt	75,150
__ 1½ oz., 3 oz. tuna fish	50,100

Vegetables

__ 6 oz., 12 oz. vegetable soup	30,60
__ 1 slice tomato, lettuce wedge	10,10
__ 6 oz., 12 oz. tossed salad	10,20

Fresh Fruit

__ ½ grapefruit	50
__ ½ orange, ½ apple	40,40
__ ½ banana	45
__ _____	
__ ½ c. canned peaches	40
__ ½ c. canned pineapple	50

Miscellaneous

__ 1 oz. diet dressing	30
__ 1 oz. diet catsup	15
__ 1 tsp. oil, 1 tsp. margarine	40,35
__ ½ bread slice	35
Total (Lunch)	C

Dinner—Menu of day

__ 5 oz. roast beef		300
__ 2 spears broccoli		20
__ salad on lettuce leaf; 5 slices cucumber; 1 onion ring		10
__ Pineapple slice w/#30 scoop cottage cheese (1 oz.)		75
	Total	405

Meat

__ 6 oz. chicken	300

Vegetables

__ 2 cucumber sticks	10

__ 1 slice tomato, lettuce wedge	10,10
__ 6 oz., 12 oz. tossed salad	10,20
__ celery or carrot sticks	10,10
__ ½ c. carrots	20
__ 2 radish roses, 2 tomato wedges, 2 celery sticks	25

Fruit

__ ½ grapefruit	50
__ ½ orange, ½ apple	40,40
__ ½ banana	45
_____	
__ ½ c. canned peaches	40
__ ½ c. canned pineapple	50

Miscellaneous

__ 1 oz. diet dressing	30
__ 1 oz. diet catsup	15
__ 1 tsp. oil, 1 tsp. margarine	40,35
__ ½ bread slice	35

Total (Dinner)   C

Total (Day)   C

EXERCISE 4—A TONER FOR FLABBY UP-PER THIGHS Lie on the floor on your right side using your right and left hands for support. Both legs should be straight out. Flex your left foot and point your toes toward your head. Then, raise your leg as high as you can with your toes still toward your head.

Start by doing this five times and add five a week until you reach twenty. After you've done the exercise on the right side, do the same on the left side five times, also adding five a week until you do twenty for each leg.

EXERCISE 5—FOR YOUR STOMACH Lie on your back with your hands behind your head. Cross your ankles. Then, bring your knees and your elbows together and touch your right elbow with your left knee. Return your feet to the floor and repeat, this time touching your left elbow with your right knee.

Start with five of each series and add five a week until you reach twenty.

EXERCISE 6—FOR YOUR STOMACH Lie on your back with your hands, palms down, underneath your buttocks. Lift your legs about six inches off the floor and keep your knees slightly bent. Do small circles with both legs simultaneously, first one way, then the other. Lower your legs and repeat. Then do the same with your legs about twelve inches off the floor. Finally do it at eighteen.

Start with five of each series and add five a week until you reach twenty.

EXERCISE 7—FOR YOUR STOMACH Lie on

your back with your legs straight and together. Put your hands behind your head and sit up using your stomach muscles for leverage. Lie back on the floor.

Start at five and work up till twenty-five by adding five sit-ups each week.

EXERCISE 8 FOR YOUR WAIST AND STOMACH Stand with your legs apart and one arm extended over your head with your palm turned away from you. Bend toward the side opposite the extended arm.

Start at ten and work up to five a week until you reach twenty-five. Then repeat with the other arm, starting at ten and working up to twenty-five.

EXERCISE 9—BUST, CHEST, AND ARMS Lie face down with your palms directly underneath your shoulders. Raise your body off the floor by extending your arms, then slowly lower yourself by bending your elbows. Push up again by straightening them. Once you have begun do not touch the floor with your body until the entire exercise is completed.

Then, push up straightening your elbows.

Women: Start with five a day and add five a week until you reach twenty-five.

Men: Start with ten a day and add ten a week until you reach forty.

EXERCISE 10—FOR ARMS AND BUST Lie on your back with arms outstretched. Get two books of equal weight and hold one with your right hand and the other with your left. Then, raise the books above your head without bending your elbows.

Repeat this ten times, adding five a week until you reach twenty-five.

And now, on to Staying Thin.

4
Why
You
Were Fat

It's said most skinny people eat to live and most fat people live to eat. But what we often fail to recognize is that the majority of fat people not only eat to live, as we all do, they also eat to *hide*.

Think back to when your weight problem was at its worst. The reason you were probably over-weight then—and the reason you kept putting the weight right back on again every time you lost it—was that deep down, *you really wanted that fat to hide behind*. Or, to put it another way, you were afraid to be thin and be forced to face the world without your protective covering.

You were using your weight to avoid facing life head on. Being fat enabled you to crawl inside your cocoon of avoirdupois and avoid problems with which you couldn't cope.

So, before you can be truly motivated to Stay Thin (not just give it lip service, but want it enough to do the type of reevaluation it requires), you must understand that no matter how obsessed you *thought* you were with getting thin, deep down you really wanted to stay fat.

Going off diets, putting on pound after pound (after you'd worked so hard to lose them), wasn't something that "just happened" to you. You *wanted* it to happen. It was something that you subconsciously chose to do, and you worked damned hard at accomplishing your goal by eating continually.

Why? Well, the world is a scary place. Each day brings new challenges: jobs, romance, confrontations of all sorts. These challenges have to be met, and they require that we present our best self to do so. Being fat is an easy cop-out, a simple way of avoiding these challenges, an excuse for not dealing with them, or dealing with them properly.

Thus, your first task is to become aware of the ways in which you have used fat to hide, used it to avoid facing the situations you find difficult and threatening. After you do that, you can work to take control of these situations, to make a concrete decision as to whether you want to come out of the fat closet and cope—or go on hiding for the rest of your life. But you can't do that until you understand why you're running away in the first place, and what you're running from.

Try this experiment. Make a list of all the people and things you find it difficult to cope with in your life. Be honest. Include all situations involving people of the opposite sex (those are often the toughest), work and job problems, skirmishes with the kids (not to mention their teachers, who can seem intimidating if you don't feel in control), irritating relatives, friends, gossipy neighbors, the man in your bank when your checkbook is overdrawn, and so on. Look long and hard at your list, and then put it away for later.

Your next step is to understand that your fat is a crutch, a ready-made excuse for your inability to rise above the petty annoyances and people in your environment. Make a conscious decision to abandon that excuse. Learn to walk without that crutch—and throw it away for good.

To do that, it may help to understand how you came to depend on that crutch in the first place. Some of my patients claimed that they know when, to one minute, they came to their turning point—in the wrong direction. Sue M., who unfortunately is still a 160-pounder, turned to food after her childhood sweetheart left her at the altar. She was so deeply hurt that she began to fear meeting other men. What if it happened again? Unconsciously, she turned to food as both solace and insurance. She began to eat and pile on the pounds; she could never be jilted a second time because she'd never be asked again.

Her problem is just a more dramatic form of a common problem among compulsive overeaters: fear of rejection. This is often allied with a fear of emotional attachments and/or sex. One of the most frequent problems I have encountered among people who have trouble maintaining

71

weight loss is their subconscious use of fat to avoid dealing with love and sex. Those who find sex threatening find fat the ideal fail-safe system for sealing themselves off from the physical world. Women don't have to deal with men. And vice versa. Sexual paranoia, on both a hetero- and homosexual level, is simply banished. Our bodies are as bland as those of Barbie and Ken dolls. For women, fear of rape disappears, along with the fear of being sexually evaluated or even accosted by the groping hands and rude looks of strangers.

Who's going to stare at you or undress you with his eyes? Nobody. Who's going to ask you out for a drink, hoping to take you off to bed, not caring a fig about who you are or what you have to say? Nobody. In fact, no one's going to look at you as a purely physical object. And, in the process, many people will probably also never bother to learn about that beautiful soul of yours. Should someone ask you for that drink, you know automatically that's *all* he wants. Which can be quite reassuring to many.

This whole area of sex more often seems to be a problem for women than for men. By being fat, a woman is able to silently declare: "I'm down on men. I don't want men to meet me so they can try to sleep with me." And once a woman gains those pounds, that usually does substantially limit her activities in the sexual arena.

But the gaining of weight to avoid sex isn't only a reaction among single women. Sometimes wives start putting on pounds at a certain point in their marriage to keep their husbands away. Occasionally, in the privacy of a medical consultation, these women still admit that they simply are no longer interested in sex, or that they want to be loved "for themselves," and not for something so superficial as the contours of their body. (Some of these same women admit, though, that they wouldn't feel very loving toward the "beautiful soul" of a big blubbery man with a spare tire around *his* waist.) And so they run away from sex by encasing themselves in protective layers of unattractive fatty tissue.

Many psychiatrists have noted that some women, deep down, somehow think that if they lose weight, they will then be free to leave an unhappy family situation. In some women this has evolved into a fantasy that if they were thinner, they'd be prettier. If they were more attractive, someone would come and take them away, and so on.

In others, it's an unarticulated feeling that if their weight changed, somehow their lives would change too. Then, when they do lose the weight, and nothing happens externally, that is, Prince Charming doesn't come along and take them away, or internally they still can't pull up their anchor and leave, for whatever reason—loyalty, guilt, lack of anyplace else to go—they rapidly put the weight back on again.

Other women get and stay fat to avoid the end products of sex: pregnancy and babies. Dottie, a devout Catholic, whose only form of birth control was the rhythm method (and she was always out of sync), began putting on weight with each pregnancy. A little here, and a little there, and pretty soon she didn't have to worry about getting pregnant any more. I guess you could call her method "girth control"—or maybe lack of it.

Some women who use fat to escape their sexuality have never known any other way. These are women who never dealt with sex, and now, at a late age, they simply don't know how. So they stay fat rather than compete in an area in which they're literally virgins. (Losing weight for them may be so terrifying that, even if it does happen, they immediately put the weight back on again.) Maybe you know a woman like that—a rotund older teacher who never married, a plain, grossly obese girl who stayed with her ailing mother instead of marrying or finding a career, etc. You rarely even see some of these folks; many are in permanent hiding.

Men get fat for some of the same reasons, but also because many fear the additional responsibility they must bear of (supposedly) having to be the dominant one in a social relationship. Even in these days of so-called women's liberation, most men still carry the primary responsibility of social intercourse—not to mention the other kind. It's still the man who is supposed to start the conversation with an unattached female, who asks for the date, who chooses the restaurant, decides the moment of the first kiss, etc. For a man who has never been in this kind of a dominant position, it can be unnerving if not downright frightening.

"Hell," admitted Tom, a patient of mine, "by the time I ordered her damn dessert I was shaking in my shoes. I knew she expected me to go with her to her apartment afterwards, but I was afraid to try. I was sure I would do something wrong and make a mess of it. So I figured I might as well order dessert for myself, too, while I was at it.''

Ease and confidence in the dating game doesn't come easily to many. And so they eat. But ironically, overcoming dating problems may lead to even more weight problems. Some who become thin, by dint of much dieting, find themselves going back to overeating and the resultant corpulence because their new life is too much for them to handle. When they lose weight, others find them more physically attractive. Meeting members of the opposite sex is easier. Getting a date is less of a hassle. They may not be able to cope with the situation emotionally—or physically. After all, you know what it's like to barely eat for a few days and then find yourself at a sumptuous buffet.

Attractive and sought after, often for the first time in their lives, they start dating a lot. They go to restaurants. They splurge on Sunday brunches. They go out drinking. And before they know it, since their bodies are as unable to handle the food situation as their minds were once unable to handle the romance, their weight starts creeping up again. Situations like this demand of these men a great deal of concentration on two principles of Staying Thin I've already mentioned: Awareness of what they're doing, and active attempts to control it.

Revenge is commonly another unconscious

motivation for being unable to Stay Thin. You often see this in marriages where both partners have lost respect for each other, can't break away, and resent being trapped. Their solution: punish the other with pounds. Overweight people who live with their parents are also sometimes seeking revenge, especially when the parents want them to be thin, or they have other expectations that the child finds it hard to live up to.

Peter, for example, moved in with his slender Park Avenue mother when his marriage—which she had engineered—broke up. Although she dined only on lean meats, vegetables, and fresh fruit in season, Peter was constantly bringing starches and rich desserts into the household. She abhorred what she called "the plebian food"—like potato chips and cellophane-wrapped cream-filled cupcakes—that he brought in, and she became equally contemptuous of Peter when he became what she considered "vulgarly fat."

When Peter finally realized that he had gotten that way to punish his mother for her interference in his activities, he also realized that allowing his midriff to go to pot (literally) just to get back at his mother was ridiculous. He moved out, slimmed down, and became a thin and socially competent person once again. But it took time.

Claudia got fat to get back at her husband and to try to make him change his ways. His job kept him out at night, and alone in their two room apartment, she ate herself into a small mountain. Her answer to him when he complained that she was getting so fat was "it's your fault. If you

76

didn't leave me alone so much, I wouldn't be bored. And if I weren't bored, I wouldn't overeat." The husband really did feel guilty about it, but he wasn't able to change his hours. Only when Claudia realized that while she was overindulging in order to get back at him the only person she was really hurting was herself was she at last able to alter her destructive eating habits.

By now you must realize that Peter, Claudia, Tom, Dottie—and you—didn't just "get fat." There was some reason that they (and you) let it happen—or subconsciously chose it to happen. The reason?

Ask *yourself* what it is for you.

Combatting your desire for calories is just a small part of your battle; combatting your subconscious need for and use of fat for protection, revenge, etc., is your strategy for winning the war.

The crucial step you must take before you can become your own Knute Rockne is: you've got to become aware of just what your problem is, to see just what you're doing to yourself. You've got to see, really see, that you're using your fat to escape from love or from life and that it just won't wash if you really want to get something out of the brief time that you're going to be in this world.

Accept it. The extra weight you've carried around has been your protection, your buffer against a hard cruel world. If you felt fragile, it made you feel solid again. The very act of eating, itself, compensated you for the loss of whatever you couldn't face: love, sex, companionship, success, whatever.

Unconsciously then, being thin, not fat, may have been your bigger problem. When you lost weight, you felt as if something had been taken away from you, and you quickly worked to regain it. Being fat was better than being scared, so you put the weight back on again.

In order to prevent that from happening again, let's look at some of the advantages you thought you had gained by being fat. That way, you can decide whether it's worth it to work to Stay Thin.

There may have been times, deep down, when you felt that being fat really wasn't that bad after all. There were probably periods when it hardly seemed worth all the effort you continually expended in order to lose weight. After all, while fat may not be beautiful in our society, it can have its selling points. Life among the legions of the obese was not bad at times—pretty comfortable, in fact.

For example, being fat took some of the anxiety out of social situations. When you were fat, there was less pressure to "be on" or perform at parties and other social gatherings. Since you were not one of the more attractive people at these events, you never had to worry about thronging admirers. Which was fine with you, since it left you more time to concentrate on the serious business at hand—eating. Being overweight also kept you from worrying about sexual rejection, since few fat people qualify as sex objects to begin with. Fat then offered you a shortcut solution to the vagaries of the interpersonal social scene—by putting you out of it completely.

Maybe you were lonely sometimes, and had no one to turn to for companionship or comfort. But food was never fickle; it was always around when you needed it. So, if you used food as a crutch, where did that leave you? Among the handicapped.

Can a handicap be an advantage—besides on a golf course? Let's look at some instances in which handicaps could indeed be a benefit. Then ask yourself, "Do you want one of your very own?"

Nobody wants to hear, for instance, that he has flat feet. But if you were a young man in 1966, it could have been better news than winning a million-dollar lottery. Why? Because it made you ineligible for the draft and kept you off the battlefield. So there are handicaps and handicaps, some of which can become very valuable under the right circumstances.

That particular war is gone. But plenty of others are still raging right now for everyone, and offering strong temptations to remain permanently 4-F in life. Like the war between the sexes, for example. I can cite hundreds of case histories attesting to the direct link between fear of sexuality and/or emotional attachments and recurring weight gain. That fear is a real handicap, and a crippling one.

But other areas besides sex are closed to the compulsive fearful fatty. Perfectly commonplace activities can be threatening if you're inexperienced, anxious, or just plain klutzy. Maybe you're one of those who want to head for the door when faced with sports and related physical activities. Even a long walk or a request to help a neighbor move a grandfather clock can trigger that old fear response. "If I helped with that clock, I'd probably drop it and smash it." "Who me? Play catch? I couldn't hit the side of the barn." "When I go for a hike I always trip over my shadow." Excuses. Excuses.

When you were hefty, you were probably just plain rotten at playing tennis and golf, the two biggest "social" sports. In fact, isn't it true that you probably never really enjoyed sports anyway, and all your life wanted excuses to duck out of invitations to play tennis, join a baseball game, or go out with the gang to bowl? Well, there was the perfect excuse, riding around your waist. How nice. How easy.

In fact, your overweight paid off for you in other ways too. On the job, or in handling business responsibilities, there were times that it was most helpful. You just couldn't take that trip to Pittsburgh. You convinced your associate to do it for you, because you were too "exhausted," although actually you simply didn't want to do all that strenuous out-of-town moving around. Or you were able to avoid meet-the-public activities like manning the company booth at a trade association convention, because chances are, when you were overweight, you weren't even asked to do it. And you knew why.

On the social scene, it was easy to beg off helping the sisterhood decorate for the church social. How could you perch on a precarious ladder and hang up streamers? Since you couldn't zip up your long dress without looking like the tubby Michelin-tire man, it was a snap to get out of

80

chaperoning at the high school prom.

So much for the social, business, and athletic scene. But those handicapping pounds didn't give you an even chance with the other players the way a golf handicap does. They kept you out of the game entirely.

And when it comes to family responsibilities, the fatty also gets out of a lot of chores because of his weight. Little League, PTA, school picnics, household tasks, all become "too much." You couldn't possibly lead the Girl Scout troop, even though Suzy begged you to, because you weren't in condition to hike around the block. Maybe you got out of the car pool because driving had become uncomfortable; you couldn't adjust the seat any further. (One of my patients said he began to feel as if he were squeezing himself into a sardine can instead of a car.) But it made you feel rotten to hear the kids snicker about you in the back seat.

And that's not all. Even your moral responsibilities took a beating. All your friends went door-to-door one week, raising money for muscular dystrophy, mental health, or some other good cause. Or they went out to pass around petitions for a new traffic light at the school crossing. But you weren't among them. Carrying all that heft around is tiring—although naturally you always gave a different excuse to others (and knew they didn't believe you).

Your body was your way out. It was your one-way ticket to indolence, to avoiding exertion and social responsibility or, for that matter, any activity you convinced yourself was not to your liking. In fact, with that excuse, you pretty much never had to do anything you didn't feel like doing.

And indeed it may have been this very laziness that helped attract you to the wrong kinds of food in the first place. Simplicity and ease are as much part and parcel of quick food and junk food as is fat. And it is these kinds of instant-gratification snacks to which most compulsive eaters gravitate. You don't have to set a table; you can eat them standing up or while seated anywhere. As naturally as breathing, they go with reading or watching TV or talking at a party. It isn't very hard work to lug along a bag of potato chips or peanuts while settling down to read the paper or watch the news.

Indeed, they're so light and portable you can carry them along in your car, to your seat in the movies, or in your pocket or handbag as you stroll around town. They don't require utensils; instead of wrestling with a knife and fork, you can just grab a handful and lift it directly to your mouth. Thus, as with everything else, even the food you chose lined the path of least resistance.

Sure, being fat was a way of avoiding exertion, but it was also a way of avoiding life. All you did was hide. Did it work well for you? Or did you really pay too high a price—forever peering over a wall of fat at the fullness of a life you couldn't live—to avoid a few uncomfortable or intimidating situations?

We all have things we'd like to hide from. Not everyone is overweight. Not everyone has chosen to turn his or her body into a living hideout. And don't think it's because others don't have your kinds of problems, because no one is immune to disappointments and hard knocks. We all have people we want to get back at—not to mention ourselves—for real or imagined slights and transgressions.

You're not the only one who is punishing himself or herself. Just add up *all* the overweight people, the smokers and the drinkers in this country alone and you've already got a population filled with people getting back at themselves and others for whatever imagined wrongs they suffered.

Now, add to those people those who suffer from other symptoms, such as workaholism (and place it high on the list); failure to dress well (whether as a matter of choice or simply not thinking or bothering to care); carelessness about personal hygiene (a casualty of our rush-rush-rush culture); drinking too much coffee or other substances best taken in moderation; not getting enough sleep; taking too many pills; etc.

The sum total: a nation of victims. Victims of needless handicaps.

Now, maybe you're one of those who subconsciously enjoys being a victim. Deep down, you like the luxury of feeling sorry for yourself. "Why shouldn't I feel sorry for myself?" Jane asked as she turned again to a high calorie security blanket. "Since my husband's accident he hasn't been able to go to work. And he's been so unpleasant to be around, that our friends won't come to see us anymore. Yet I have to spend all my time caring for an injured, surly person. He certainly has no feelings for me, so I have them for myself.''

Give some thought to what you've *really* gained by being fat and what you've lost on account of it. Think of why you really let yourself get that way. What were you trying to avoid? Who were you trying to punish—beside yourself?

Do you really want to go through life buying clothes at special stores, and looking longingly (but hopelessly) at the glamorous garb in boutique windows? Or having people stare at you when you reach for a third helping in a restaurant—and return for the umpteenth time to the smorgasbord? Or watching others strut around in bikinis at the beach, while you cover up in a sweatshirt or a robe? Or do you want to spend your whole life standing around at parties while you and the Mallomars become an item?

For one thing, how do you think you looked to others then? Maybe you've convinced yourself that you were really not that unattractive when you looked like a balloon. Forget it. If anyone ever told you that you looked better fat than thin, you probably shouldn't trust them.

There's only one place you can safely put your trust: the mirror. Take off all your clothes. Turn on the bright lights. And look.

Would you look better—or worse— if you took off more pounds? Did you look better when you weighed much more than you do now? So much for the physical advantages of fat.

No, there's no way to make fat a winner. No

way to change the fact that we admire thinness, we advertise it, publicize it, glamorize it, validate it and reward it every way we know how.

As a result, sooner or later—usually sooner—the overeater starts to feel like a confirmed criminal, a repeater, walking around guilt-ridden after each antisocial act. You feel as if every finger is pointing at you, that everyone knows you for what you are, and hates you for it. So what do you do? Pull out a bag of potato chips, go off in the corner—and eat.

In the end, a happy fat person is a contradiction in terms. We overeat because we are unhappy, dissatisfied with our lives. What better way to divert ourselves from our problems than by devoting our energies to systematic overeating. But it's the kind of therapy guaranteed to make you hate yourself—and you don't have to wait for the morning after.

Most of the people you've been reading about weren't aware of the ways in which they were using their fat to get what they wanted—or get back at whom they wanted. Once you figure out what it is you're doing, once you gain awareness of your manipulative tactics, you're halfway down the road to change and control

If Peter had realized, for instance, that although he was eating to punish his mother, he was actually the one taking the punishment, he could have changed his ways much more quickly. (By becoming aware of his problems, he did finally gain control.) Or a chubby secretary, munching potato chips and nibbling at the gumdrops she hides in her desk drawer, was aware that she fears a promotion and the new responsibilities it would entail, she could face her fears of inadequacy and use her awareness to help gain control of her life. And that's when the scales would start to dip.

Yes, there's hope for everyone. The deserter can become the decorated general and lead the troops into victory. The fatties can start to live again—once they realize that that's what they want to do.

Do you want to stop being a victim? A handicapped person? Someone running away from the opposite sex, someone getting back at themselves in the belief that they're getting back at another, some running away from life itself?

Wouldn't you really rather Stay Thin?

5
Why
You Want
to Stay Thin

Hopefully, by now you're at the point where you're giving your figure, your wardrobe, and your former fatty lifestyle a few not-too-nostalgic backward glances. "Being fat," says Gloria F., a textile designer, "locked me into a way of life as effectively as a jail sentence. There were so many rules and restrictions and limitations, I could practically hear the keys jangle. Now that I'm out of my padded cell—pun intended—I'll never go back to jail again!"

Staying Thin will help you to find yourself, and free yourself from having food as your main focus. You'll start living for more in life than just your next meal, and as a result, others will find you more interesting. Being fat kept you from developing as a person and realizing your full potential. It also isolated you from the rest of the world—except for fat people like yourself.

"Now," confides Jean L., "I can really find out who *I* am and what I like to do. Before, my whole life was organized around food. Most of my friends were fatties too. Now, I'm finding that people react to me, not my weight, to what I think and feel, and to how I express myself. And it feels good."

Sports are something else that may open up for you once you keep that weight off. Ed M. at 280 was so lazy that his friends used to kid him by suggesting that he would have taken a cab to the incinerator if he possibly could. Now, at 180, he has discovered that since he no longer has to carry an extra hundred pounds along with him, he really enjoys running.

Getting interested in sports has opened up some social horizons for him as well. "There's more than one zoo in Central Park," he laughed. "The whole place is like a zoo—at mating season. And the girls who jog are all good-looking." Well, at least they're sure to be thin. Fat people (male or female) usually don't jog; it's embarrassing and it's too difficult, so you rarely see the potbellies and the balloon thighs on the jogging track.

Staying Thin also frees you from some of your fears about diseases. After all, being fat is not only a bummer, but as I stated earlier, it's also a killer. Obesity leads to—or complicates—all kinds of medical conditions such as major diseases of the heart and arteries (including arteriosclerosis, high blood pressure, angina pectoris, varicose veins, etc.), diabetes, cirrhosis, kidney disease, even arthritis.

Not surprisingly, weight control is considered to be one of the most effective measures available to prevent or delay the onset of the major degenerative diseases, as well as to extend the length of your active useful life. Any doctor or insurance company will tell you that a thin person is at once less likely to fall prey to dieases and better able to throw off infection. (Thin people are also less prone to accidents, which makes them better insurance risks in general.)

And yet ironically, many overweight people truly believe that they're healthier than the thin folks. This myth may stem from childhood, since so many of them were brought up in families where a plump child was considered a healthier child. A patient of mine, Simon S., recalls that his mother "was constantly worried about my sister, Lillian, who was so thin she looked like you could break her in two. So how come Lillian has hardly ever been sick in her life, while I have to take blood pressure medication for the rest of my life?" he asked.

The erroneous child-rearing notion that chubby is healthy and thin is sick often carries over to our present-day lives. "Every time I lose a little weight," complains Shirley H, "I catch a cold or I start to feel weak and dizzy. Then I get afraid that all this dieting is going to make me sick, or anemic or something, so I start eating again."

Just as people say they feel sick if they diet and use that as an excuse to start eating again, so also do people use genuine sickness as an excuse to do what they want—overeat. "If I get a cold when I'm dieting," says Annette C., "I feel like I have to drink a lot of orange juice, drink chicken soup, and have several pieces of toast. Bang. There goes my diet." (Actually, you don't need to "stuff a cold," as grandmother would say. Vitamin supplements, proper medical attention, and adequate rest should be sufficient.)

Keep in mind that being or becoming thin does not make you unhealthy; being or becoming fat does. There are too many insurance studies to even enumerate which prove that you're unlikely to live as long if you're a fatty—and we all know that those last years, sick and fat, won't be much to write home about either.

Furthermore, obese people generally have higher medical expenses. Aside from their proneness to fatigue and degenerative diseases, they just don't seem to feel very well a lot of the time. Their insurance premiums also cost them more (obesity is a risk), and they seem to have to go to all kinds of doctors that thin people can skip—nutritionists, varicose vein specialists, or bariatric doctors like myself.

Another area in which it pays to be thin is employment. One of my patients, Randy S., is in the employment agency business. He says that "when overweight people come into the agency to be interviewed for possible job openings, I speak right up and tell them that employers are reluctant to hire obese people. This is not a matter of discrimination, as fat people are apt to suspect.

Nor is it a matter of aesthetic consideration. The companies' insurance simply won't cover obese people.''

Randy also faces the issue of appearance squarely and realistically. "When I call an employer to recommend a client, the employer asks often about the client's personal appearance. I tell the truth; if the client is a slob, or has stringy hair and dirty fingernails, I mention it. If he or she is fat, I mention that, too. Frankly, it doesn't produce a very enthusiastic response.''

No matter how you look at it, or what your "sexual politics" are, there's no way of denying that a thin person makes a better first impression than does a fat one. Most interviews are conducted sitting down; the interviewer faces the applicant. There's no way of avoiding that all-emcompassing stare. Rolls around the middle, bulging hips, trouser legs bursting at the seams, ankles that won't cross—nobody likes to look at these; and nobody fails to notice them, though they might might pretend otherwise.

The Equal Opportunity legislation doesn't say that it's illegal to discriminate against fat people— and believe me, employers do.

As we said before, it's not only appearance that causes this discrimination; characterological fat has connotations too. When others see fat people they assume, sometimes wrongly but more often correctly, that they aren't in control. If they can't control their weight, others wonder, how they can be expected to be punctual, well-organized, well-balanced and emotionally reliable? Discrimina-

91

tion? Maybe so. But it's better to avoid it altogether than to try to battle so pervasive a prejudice.

On the flip side, a good, trim appearance will do worlds for your chances at that new job and for promotion in your current one. A look of "having it all together"—a trim body, clothes that fit, nice accessories—gives the impression that you can cope, and that is what employers are looking for.

Yes, thin is definitely *in* in business. One study showed (though one hardly needs a study to prove something so obvious!) that of two salesmen, one weighing 180 pounds and the other weighing 250, people bought the product from guess who.

As for getting the job in the first place, whom do you think the personnel manager chooses if two candidates are equally qualified but one of them is fat? Put yourself on the other side of the desk. Which one would you choose?

And what if you were thin when you got the job, but as the years accumulated, so did the pounds? That can mean never getting your name on the door or the carpeting on the floor, or getting stuck at a salary level that just won't support your present lifestyle. Or, to be more gloomy about it, you might even lose your job altogether.

We all know that models (and racetrack jockeys) can't gain even a pound without risking their careers. But even in situations that aren't that clear-cut, fat people's careers suffer because of their weight. Today's corporations are looking for people who can cut a good figure with the public. And while it's true that the president of the corporation himself may be overweight, he probably was not that way on his way up.

Studies have shown that obese people have lower paying jobs—for the reason I've just mentioned—and yet, life costs more for the overweight. There's no question that food costs more. But clothes do too, since manufacturers can charge more for a size fifty-eight suit than a five.

Marianne P. gets around this dilemma by making her own clothes, but she realizes that they're shapeless and unattractive. Furthermore, she has learned that there are some things—like bras and pantyhose—that she can't make and that are next to impossible to buy or have custom-made when you're fat.

Another patient, Judi D., thinks she has solved her problem by wearing caftans all the time. Even when Judi goes to the beach in the summer, she wears a tasteful terrycloth caftan. She has them all made for her by a dressmaker, and the fabrics are beautiful and the detailing exquisite. Even so, she invariably looks like an elephant dressed by Omar the Tentmaker, and she's really fooling no one.

Thin people, on the other hand, seem to be able to wear almost anything (or almost nothing) and get away with it. "I used to buy long-skirted, one-piece bath suits to hide my blubbery legs and rolling tummy," says Selma H. "But now that I'm thin, I can improvise. Last summer I made a bikini out of three thirty-nine cent bandannas from the five and dime store. My sixteen-year-old daughter liked it so much she actually borrowed it from me. You can imagine how good that made me feel. Not only was I saving money and feeling creative, but I was getting compliments instead of embarrassed stares from the critical younger generation."

So far we've only been talking about the average overweight person. But really obese people have truly *tremendous* problems with expenses. Some must travel first class on planes because they need the wider space in the seat. Some are too fat to get behind the wheel of a small foreign car, and must either buy a big American car or take taxis everywhere they go. Getting around is literally a big problem. They could, and probably should, walk more often, but their excess weight is a pain to drag around, and they're prone to shortness of breath.

On the other hand, thin people can have great pleasure getting from place to place on their own power—walking, jogging, biking in the city; cross-country skiing and snowshoeing; even horseback riding. A fatty on a horse is something else!

So, being fat can make you sick, or even kill you; it can keep you in a low-paying, no-growth job; it can and most often does ruin your social life; and it can cost you the money you haven't been able to earn because you've been sick and/or stuck in that crummy job, and so fat you couldn't climb the ladder of success without breaking a couple of the rungs.

Who needs it?

But almost no one is going to make the enormous effort to Stay Thin permanently just because of the dangers in, and the destructive results of, allowing oneself to stay fat. The avoidance of something negative isn't enough to motivate such a long-haul endeavor. People require intensively positive motivation to provide the extra push they need to make that Thin-for-Life decision—and stick to it.

So look back at that list I asked you to make of people and situations you found it difficult to cope with. Now, imagine yourself twenty pounds thinner (and wearing a new outfit which you know you won't outgrow). Think of yourself at your best. Imagine that you have complete confidence in your ability to handle these problems. How many of those situations still seem scary? Sure, some will. No one claims that a thin figure solves all of life's difficulties. But I'll bet some of the items on that list would seem considerably less ominous if you confront them looking and feeling your very best.

Now, make a list of all the positive things you could really enjoy if you were looking and feeling your best, a list of reasons for wanting to look and feel wonderful. Start with the situations you encounter at home and in your personal life, and then go on to job and professional situations, dealing also with petty annoyances in all areas—bank tellers, grouchy plumbers, snippy salespeople.

Do your reasons have to do with your job? Your marriage? Your hobbies? Do you imagine an end to awkwardness on the tennis court? An end to embarrassment in the bedroom? An upsurge of confidence at the board meetings?

A few goodies that will crop up on everyone's list (just to help you along) are enjoying yourself at parties, relaxing in restaurants, buying whatever clothes you like (without concern about weight), *and* looking good in them, eating your favorite dish for the pleasure of it, not out of a compulsion to, having freedom from fear of degenerative diseases, moving with ease in crowded rooms, trains, not to mention those narrow aisles in airplanes, and those are just starters.

How about the relief of never being ashamed of your body—of disrobing easily in the doctor's office, of walking freely down the beach, of making love with the light on, or of feeling just like anyone else in the communal try-on room of discount clothes stores. Just think of the pleasure of looking in a full-length mirror, even under fluorescent lights, and thinking "Wow" instead of "Yuk."

Look in your closets and list all the satisfactions that have to do with clothing. Check out your address book and your appointment calendar. Slip behind the wheel of your car (or step up into a bus, or squeeze into a crowded subway). Extend your list to include rewards at the office, among your friends and peers. Back at your desk, look at your checkbook and your bank balance. Being thin is going to save you money. Count the ways.

List the little reasons too. Like leaning over to pat the cat without feeling a bulge hanging over your waistband. *Everything* you can think of in favor of getting and Staying Thin.

And if you're a parent, ask your kids why they'd like to see you Stay Thin. They'll tell you—unfortunately. Kids have a very unflattering, and brutally frank, vocabulary for describing all the ills of adults, and fat is no exception. Wouldn't it be nice to be immune from that forever?

But the best reason may be the last entry written by a patient in one of our groups. Her final reason was that "you can never be too rich or too thin." When I asked her how that could be a specific reason for Staying Thin, she countered by saying that "I have lots of specific reasons as you can see from the rest of my list. But the bottom line is to hell with all the reasons: I just want to be thin."

Yes, that's the way you can be, and you can have the feeling of freedom from constraint, of being in control, and of not being at the mercy of anything or anyone, be it a domineering mother, or an intimidating boss, or a box of cookies, or a lunchtime martini. Remember this: if you're motivated enough to work at it, every weight problem has a solution.

Yours is within your reach.

6
How Your
Compulsive Eating
Began

Now that we've talked about why you shouldn't overeat, and why you should control your eating habits, let's turn to one of the reasons why you actually do the forbidden deed.

Most of you, no doubt, are "repeat offenders." You "do your time," lose weight, "go straight" for a while, and then go back to your criminal activity—overeating—thereby putting yourself right back in prison again.

You know it's not rational. You know it doesn't make sense. You know it's wrong. But just like the habitual criminal, the overeater doesn't really understand his motives. You know you shouldn't do it, but you do it again and again. You are driven.

But if you become aware of what drives you,

you don't have to be driven to the fathouse any more. So first, let's look at what that drive actually is and what being driven really means.

Compulsive behavior is doing something to excess because you can't help it. In most instances, people who are driven to perform, or to consume, or even to talk about something compulsively choose an object that is—to use an old cliché—either illegal, immoral, or fattening. Kleptomaniacs steal, arsonists set fires, alcoholics drink, and fatties eat.

Those people are not in control of their actions. Most sincerely wish they could stop, and many—like some shoplifters who steal items they don't even want or need—are hardly aware that they're doing it.

Think about some of the minor compulsions you and people you know have. We all know someone who compulsively empties the ashtrays the moment a guest finishes a cigarette, plumps the pillows the instant someone gets up from the couch, or washes his or her hands fifty times a day. Other common examples are nail-biting, eternally making lists, twisting a strand of hair around one's fingers (or tying it into a knot), always checking the mailbox twice to make sure the letters went down, etc. These are harmless, mildly annoying forms of compulsive behavior.

But when such behavior involves putting something into your mouth, there's an added dimension to the compulsiveness. Not only is it usually out of control, but the person with the compulsion is also most likely damaging their body by filling it with an excess of some substance that probably isn't good for it in the first place.

Why do you have this compulsion to do that?

WHAT CRAVERS CRAVE

How many overweight people do you know (yourself included) who binge on carrot sticks? Celery? Even fruit (though that can cause an enormous weight gain if eaten in excess)? None. Usually compulsive eaters choose foods that are high in starch or sugar. Some of the worst offenders gorge on potato chips, cakes, cookies, candy, nuts, and soft drinks.

Why do people crave these particular foods and eat them repeatedly, day in and day out? Is it hunger? Is our system honestly begging us for Fritos? Or does that food that we compulsively consume, on a habitual basis, stand for something else? FOOD IS LOVE. No one's overlooking the fact that we eat to live; to nourish ourselves adequately, we must take in calories, proteins, vitamins, etc. But that doesn't explain why we prefer one food to another, sometimes to the point of gross overindulgence. Pascal once wrote, "The heart has its reasons which reason knows nothing of." That's true also of the stomach.

Food and our emotions are intertwined from the very beginning of our existence. From the first drops of milk down a newborn baby's throat, it learns that food is love. If it's fed enough, and at the right time, it feels loved. If it isn't fed when it's hungry, more than its body goes unnourished: Lack of food is lack of love.

Growing up, and as an adult, it will try to make up for that lack. There are other ways to compensate for real and imagined childhood deprivation, but the fastest, easiest, and most direct way is to overeat. And since we live in a society where food is overabundant, overadvertised, overemphasized, and overritualized, it's natural that we turn to it as our primary solace.

Many of my patients have told me that their mothers, following old-fashioned child-rearing practices, claim they fed them on four-hour schedules. Hunger may have set in after three hours, but no matter; the schedule was strictly adhered to. When they grew up, these people became overeaters to try to satisfy those long-ago hungers.

You may be like them, or, more likely, you may suffer from a different kind of "food is love" mix-up: the "love is food" kind. When adults wanted to show you that they loved you, they stuffed you with sweet things like cookies, cakes, lollipops, whatever. Whether or not you were hungry.

Another thing many of you had in common was a grandmother who was in charge of the kitchen. Every time Rosemary M. did well in school, her fat Italian grandmother rewarded her with a goody. Every time Martin B. hurt himself, his fat Jewish grandmother gave him a treat to salve the wound.

Although in most cases grandmother is no longer with us—or else she's slim and trim and offering us yogurt and raw vegetables these days—she's still left a small voice inside many of her grandchildren, urging them to "eat, eat."

It would be so easy to listen to that voice and be a child again, loved despite (or perhaps because) of your hefty body. Thus, some people overeat to rekindle and recapture the long lost childhood feeling of being loved and cared for once again. Perhaps that's been your problem too.

Most likely food in your family was also used as a pacifier. Whether you had an unhappy overstuffed childhood or not, whether or not there was a grandma-temptress in your kitchen, or a food faddist, or someone who exercised too rigid a control over the icebox, you learned soon enough that food was a way to make you feel better, an easy way to cope with distress.

Unfortunately, the "lollipop principle" is still with us. When a pediatrician gives a shot, or a barber cuts a child's hair, doesn't he frequently offer candy afterwards to sweeten the ordeal?

The truth is, food was and is an extremely effective pacifier. Florence K. recalls taking her six-month-old baby on their first airplane trip together. The baby started fussing the minute the plane took off, but was instantly soothed when a stewardess opened a packet of sugar and trickled it into his mouth. "He had never tasted anything like it," Florence reports. "He was stunned by the wonderfulness of it. He looked like he was thinking 'This is what heaven must be like.' "

Louisa L. remembers the car trips her family took back and forth to their weekend house in the country, when she and her brothers and sisters were young. "When we got restless, or started to whine and fuss, mother would pass out the goodies and we would get quiet. When I got older, and began driving long distances myself, I had a tough time breaking the nibble habit in the car."

Other eating habits instilled in our youths may lead us to rebel with completely opposite behavior later on: vegetables first, dessert later; if you hate something, take at least three bites of it anyway; come to the table promptly and sit through the entire meal, etc. Many children, who have been brought up this way, rebel later against the organized eating habits their families insisted upon by becoming rabidly informal about food. They eat in bed, or in the middle of the night, or standing up, or in the car, etc. Such "methodically" casual eating does not lend itself to meals of vegetables, yogurt, and lean meats. It cries out for fast food, junk food, sweet food, takeout food, and most especially the kinds of things that come wrapped up: cupcakes, candy bars, cookies, etc.

It's true that some children who were forced to clean their plates, or who were overindulged with food, managed to grow up thin in spite of it all. But it's more likely that you're one of those who got tubby early, wore "chubby" or "husky" sizes from an early age, and never even thought about being any other way.

A typical example is Ellen C., who was not only fat, but also wore glasses at a time when few children did. "I'll never forget the chanting of my schoolmates: 'Fatty, fatty, two-by-four. Can't get through the bathroom door.'

103

"They called me 'fatso four eyes,' " she continued sadly, still to this day hurt by those memories. "It never occurred to me that I could change. I felt so terrible that I used to come home from school and eat and eat." And her mother didn't try to stop her. In fact, she encouraged Ellen's gorging, and was waiting at the door with a plate of cookies when Ellen came home from school, crying. Obviously she thought that was love.

Many mothers (and sometimes fathers not to mention grandparents) made matters much worse, either by overestimating or underestimating the weight problem. During those terrible teens, did your mother tell you that you were beautiful—when you were really badly overweight? Or did she go in the other direction and tell you things like you were too fat to ever catch a mate?

It's been said in talking about ghetto youth, that if you tell a boy often enough that he's going to become a thief, sooner or later he'll oblige you by turning into one. It's also true that if you tell someone frequently enough that he/she is no good, unattractive, and definitely not charming, special or brilliant, the time will come when he or she will oblige you by fulfilling your negative prophecies. If your mother convinced you that you were fat and unattractive, you may have decided there was nothing you could do about it and it was your fate to grow up still fat and unattractive.

But you can't sit around now and blame your parents (or grandparents) for making you fat.

Doing that accomplishes nothing, and it is highly likely to make you eat more. Just remember that they had their problems too. Overeating in teenagers is hard to handle because teenagers are hard to handle. It requires tact and understanding, not nagging. And you were probably one of many whose parents didn't realize that.

It's easy to see that most childhood eating problems can be traced to parents, not only through what they fed their child physically but also emotionally. Parents, and grandparents, unwittingly foist their own food compulsions (along with everything else) on to their children—and thus the bad eating habits are started and perpetuated.

Studies have shown that a child will naturally eat what's right if he/she is given the opportunity to do so. A. S. Neill, the noted (and controversial) British educator, found that "any mother can set out on a table ice cream, candy, whole-wheat bread, tomatoes, lettuce, and other foods, and then allow the child complete freedom to eat what he wants. The average child, if not interfered with, will select a balanced diet."

Children are not naturally junk food addicts, any more than they are naturally smokers, drinkers, or criminals. You didn't come out of the womb crying out for a Yoo-Hoo or some Frito-Lays. All these habits are learned.

And learned behavior can be modified. There's no reason why, just because you developed bad eating habits as a child, or confused the meaning of food and this stayed with you as an adult, that you can't change your behavior now. Most people with your kind of weight problems had your kind of problems early on too. But many have been able to conquer them and Stay Thin.

And you can too.

7
Bingeing:
The Beginning
of the End

Consider bingeing. It's a lone adventure. There are no pointing fingers to spoil the pleasure. No accusing eyes to watch. And just as people slink off by themselves to indulge in other acts that make them feel guilty—masturbation, reading pornography, whatever—bingers slink off alone to indulge in their insatiable craving for food.

They pad downstairs in slippers and softly open the refrigerator door for a midnight snack. And then they let go as an out-of-town conventioneer hundreds of miles from home might do with a lady. But here there's no infidelity to a spouse; only infidelity to one's body. In their solitude, with no one to accuse or laugh, with their conscience banked or at least turned down low, bingers can kick up their heels and go hog-wild.

Which they do. Once again, the bingers become children, doing whatever they want, permitting themselves no real thought of the consequences.

Most people with weight problems have learned life's early lessons too well. They turn to food when they need love. They turn to food when they need to be pacified. They turn to food when their lives go wrong. They eat whether or not they're hungry because it is not hunger they are responding to. They are eating in response to their emotions at that time.

A lot of people don't want to believe that their feelings can have so much power over them. "I'm from Missouri," says Louise J. "You have to show me." O.K., Louise; let's show you.

I'll start by telling you about some rats. These weren't gaunt, hungry, garbage-can raiders, but well-fed tenants of a University of Pittsburgh laboratory. They earned their keep by working in a psychology experiment. When the rats' tails were pinched (lightly) they went on eating binges.

Now tails have little, if anything, to do with stomachs and hunger. Why should a rat, feeling his tail being pinched, overindulge at mealtimes? Because the pinch made him anxious. And because the food was there.

If a piece of wood were there instead, an anxious rat might gnaw it. If another rat had been there, a nervous rat might have behaved aggressively or sexually. But these other outlets were not available to them—only the extra food was—so overeating was what 95 percent of the approximately 4,000 rats tested turned to whenever they became anxious.

Is this beginning to remind you of something?

Another thing about these rats: they didn't just overeat; they became compulsive overeaters. Eventually, when their tails were pinched, they even preferred eating—remember, they weren't hungry to begin with—to mating. They had learned to overeat as a response to the anxiety-provoking tail-pinching.

Now what does this mean for you and me? Scientists are a cautious group. They don't like to draw conclusions until all the facts have been garnered. But I think we can safely assume that these rats have learned to overeat in order to distract themselves from their feelings of pain and anxiety.

And I think we can recognize too that, as human beings, we are also tempted to turn to food when we're anxious or under stress—like the rats. We taught ourselves (or were taught, most likely by our parents or grandparents) to turn to food when we are anxious, unhappy, need to be pacified, need to feel we are loved, etc.

Furthermore, this is true at all ages. A teenage patient recently conducted a study of her own senior class. Since she was studying the problems of stress, she prepared a questionnaire to coincide with the time the seniors were waiting to get their acceptances—or rejections—from the colleges. Many of the students listed symptoms of irritability, bad dreams, frequent urination, forget-fulness, and other classic signs of tension during this period.

But the overwhelming majority confessed to overeating. "I gained five pounds in a week," one girl admitted. "I chain-chewed Life Savers," revealed another. "I would come home from school, and just stand at the open-refrigerator door, ruminating. Since my apartment was badly air-conditioned, I actually convinced myself I was doing it to get cool," said a third student. But for all of them, it's easy to guess how this stressful situation affected them: in pounds.

And it's also easy to see how grownups, with often even more stress in their lives—a divorce, a new job, money problems, a battle with a teen-age son, a senile parent, an alcoholic spouse—could also turn to the refrigerator.

Studies have shown that the overweight person has more difficulty than the nonobese in discriminating the hunger signal from their other body signals and needs, including emotional ones. A person without a weight problems says "I am hungry" when true physiological sign signals of hunger beckon. But many of those with weight problems say the same thing when what they are in fact experiencing are emotional signals of anxiety, depression, stress, fear, etc. The result is an inability to Stay Thin, no matter how successfully they occasionally diet, until they realize what they're really doing.

For example, Jeff was a harried businessman who couldn't make ends meet, no matter how much time he spent working. Whenever he felt overwhelmed or frustrated by his financial situation, which happened several times a day, he interpreted the vague feeling of frustration as hunger, and turned to snacks for solace.

Ellen, a graduate student in psychology, thought that impending exams for some physiological reason, made her ravenously hungry. But what was really happening was that toward the end of every semester, her work would pile up, exams for which she was unprepared would loom ahead, and she would become anxious. Mild anxiety, often experienced as slight nervousness or queasiness, is very commonly misinterpreted as hunger and consequently misdirected into an urge to splurge—on food.

Poor Jack. Every day his boss would point out errors in his work, even though the boss himself made a large number of serious boners. But naturally Jack couldn't comment on *them*. So Jack's anger festered, and he began to increase his after-lunch walks to a nearby shopping center. At such times, he would invariably "feel hungry"— and I don't have to tell you the rest.

Don had a problem that is commonly misconstrued as craving for food: sexual frustration. After what he thought was a happy marriage of sixteen years, he could no longer deny to himself that his wife had no further interest in sex whatsoever. Nonetheless, he kept trying. Sometimes he was rebuffed altogether; sometimes his wife would perfunctorily perform the sex act, which often made him feel even worse than when he was turned away. Either way, he would leave the bedroom afterwards and wander down to the kitchen, where a "craving for food" came over him, even though he had usually finished a full dinner just a few hours earlier.

Might the same thing that happened to them have happened to you?

EATING—THE WRONG RESPONSE

Like the rats, we learned to overeat when we are upset, often because we've confused hunger with craving. But since overeating is a learned behavior pattern, it can therefore be unlearned. To do this, though, you have to understand why you established the wrong behavior pattern in the first place.

Throughout your life, you've gone on one diet or another. Some of them have worked for a while and your weight went down. But whenever problems came along, you had the same old wrong response—you ate—and soon your weight bounced right back up again.

Think back to some heavy problem periods in your life, when you also overate. Did eating really help you to finally solve those problems? And when you lost weight, and became distressed over some petty disturbances, did going off your diet make your daily troubles disappear? For instance, you might have reached your "magic number," 113 lbs., or whatever it was, and your mother *still* called you on the phone daily with her petty grievances. Your youngest child *still* got into trouble in school. Your spouse *still* had a hard time getting along with his boss and came home grumpy and sour. Turning to food for comfort, and for assistance in handling these day-to-day crises, accomplished nothing. Nor will it in the future.

You had better accept the fact right now that while your pounds may leave you, your problems will not. When you felt sorry for yourself, and went slinking off to the refrigerator, there was no help for your problems inside it. All you did was create more problems for yourself. One of the hardest lessons on learning to Stay Thin is to come to fully accept the fact that food is *never* a solution to *any* problem.

One of the most unhappy situations any of my patients has gone through while dieting was when one man learned that his father's leg was about to be amputated. Now there's no doubt that's a pretty upsetting situation to be in. And you might argue that *anything* that made him feel better at a time like that—like eating a lot of his favorite foods—was O.K.

But would overeating *really* have made him feel any better? Think back to how guilty you felt after the last time you binged. The pleasure of the food in your mouth lasted only a few minutes. The guilt and self-reproach lasted for hours, sometimes even days. And the weight itself remained for months.

No, eating never solved anyone's problems, including yours. The brutal fact about this man's situation was that, whether or not he overate, his father's condition would still be the same. Even if he binged on ten pounds of food in one sitting, his father's leg would still have to be amputated. And he would have felt just as bad about it as if he had

had only a cup of strong tea with no sugar.

By now, it certainly should be apparent to you that eating, in response to anything but genuine hunger, is the *wrong* response. Eating as a substitute for love, or as a way to handle negative emotions or personal crises, doesn't work. You can eat and eat. Do you feel more loved after bingeing? Are you happy and cheerful instead of miserable and blue? Have any of your problems miraculously vanished?

Many people turn to food as if it were a magic elixir. And in many ways, it *is* magical. Eating is a diversion; it takes your mind off your troubles. It offers instant—albeit temporary—pleasure, in contrast to the pain and anxiety which, in a serious and long-term crisis, never seems to abate. It's also often a social activity, a way to avoid the loneliness that surrounds most of our lives.

But like much magic, a curse often goes along with it. This kind of "short-order" therapy can only mask your problems—not solve them. And in the long run, it will even add to them.

If you are undergoing a truly dire personal crisis, you would do well instead of overeating to seek professional help, whether from a therapist, clergyman, or social worker. If therapy is out of the question, try to spend as much time as possible talking about the crisis and expressing your feelings about it to a friend, a relative, or someone with whom you feel close.

Many people—particularly men—feel that it's stronger, more mature, and more admirable to keep their troubles bottled up inside them. Terry B., for example was such a person. When his wife of nineteen years walked out on him, he suffered the proverbial broken heart, but he kept on going and outwardly displayed his usual cheerful disposition. Colleagues at his office, his relatives, and even his close friends were amazed at how little anguish he showed. He just never talked about his wife. But gradually, they began to notice something else: Terry, always a trim man, was developing a paunch and a double chin.

"I didn't realize it at the time," he told me later, "but my eating habits completely changed. Instead of a regular dinner waiting for me, there'd be an empty refrigerator. So I would go out for pizza. I bought cakes too, along with pastries and donuts for breakfast. I began to snack at my desk during the day—a bag of potato chips, a Coke— teen-age food. It just crept up on me."

So did the weight. Terry had a hard time getting his weight back down again and establishing independent eating patterns. But at the same time, at my advice, he began having regular talks with one of his old friends who was also in the process of a divorce. Talking about his problems reduced his stress, and that helped diminish his craving for the sweets he needed to satisfy him. In that way, he helped his emotional state as well as his midriff. Reducing his eating also made him feel that he was accomplishing something rather than doing something destructive. And, as a side effect, his increased mastery over food brought him a confidence that made him better able to handle his personal crisis.

There is only one kind of crisis in which to continue dieting and attempting to Stay Thin may not be advisable. If someone is severely depressed, possibly even suicidal, depriving him of that "fast, fast, fast relief" offered by his favorite foods may be dangerous. But even while such a person is overeating to solve his problems (which it won't), he should place himself under a doctor's care, preferably a specialist in emotional problems. It's possible that in time and with some therapy, they won't feel any further need to resort to food as stopgap therapy.

UNHAPPINESS THAT CAN
LEAD TO BINGEING

It's not only specific problems or immediate crises that lead us to binge. There are times when life seems to be going along pretty smoothly, we can't complain, we can't pinpoint any serious situations that are disturbing us, and yet we have a relapse. The precipitating factor is often a general feeling of malaise; a sense of unhappiness without knowing the exact reason for it. We may not have the feeling all the time; just often enough to lead us to the refrigerator door at unexpected moments and always for inordinate amounts of food. For some, this happens at specific times, like midnight; for others, the urge can strike at any time.

In order to fight those special moments, when something "comes over you" which leads you to overeat, you have to recognize that something *is* coming over you and that something has nothing

116

to do with hunger. If you don't recognize that your tail is being pinched, that is, that you are undergoing anxiety, unhappiness, etc., you may think that you are responding to hunger, or you may react (overeating) without really being aware of what you're doing at all. And many of us don't really recognize when we're feeling unhappy unless we have a tangible external problem we can blame everything on.

But unhappiness is often present just below the surface, and it includes feelings that range from acute agony, to sheer misery, to chronic discontent, to just plain old boredom. Often you are so out of touch with your feelings that although you may recognize that you're unhappy, you have no idea of the reason for it. There may even be times when you are so out of touch with yourself that you don't even realize that you're feeling down. (Some people talk about blue as if it were a color.) Doesn't it make sense that once you understand that you are overeating in response to a particular negative feeling, you can work to eliminate that feeling, or at least devise a better type of response to it?

KINDS OF UNHAPPINESSES— AND WAYS TO HANDLE THEM

Let's look at some typical kinds of unhappiness that can turn you to food for comfort.

For a starter, bad eating habits can come into play when you are bored. (Many psychologists believe that boredom is in fact a mask for anxiety anyway, but that's another matter.) Perhaps you are studying for a big exam. Apathy has settled over you like a heavy fog. In your state of peak restlessness, you begin to nibble. And nibble. And nibble—until you find yourself surrounded by the debris of your binge.

The same thing is likely to happen when we're frustrated. Frustration is one of the commonest kinds of unhappiness, and the way we respond to it is often self-defeating. George R.'s problem, for instance, was frustration with his job. He wasn't rising in his company and others who were hired after him were being promoted over him. One mark against him, as George was finally able to recognize, was his near 300-pound bulk. It's very unusual, as we discussed earlier, for fat people to succeed in business.

By giving in to his feelings of frustration and "going crazy" in the kitchen, George was actually one of the main causes of his own lack of success. Now, when that "Mr. Hyde" feeling comes along, George puts on his hat and coat and goes out for a walk. This gets him away from his kitchen, and also works off a few calories as well. He has also learned—the hard way after one disastrous walk past a bakery—not to bring any money with him when he's off on his perambulations.

Now, no one can promise George that he'll become president of his company. As he loses weight, however, and as he continues to keep it off, his self-confidence will increase and, as a result, so will other people's confidence in him. So far, George has lost about twenty-five pounds. Every pound marks a gain in his self-confidence.

I'll bet that soon he'll be able to walk past that bakery with a pocket full of money, and not spend a dime.

Feeling down, or mildly depressed, is another form of unhappiness, and a very insidious one. "I don't know why," some of my patients complain, "but I just feel low." So they give themselves that "quick fix," high calorie food that physically they don't really even want. And guess what? It makes them feel even lower.

Guilt is another problem that commonly leads to bingeing. Nobody is so pure and innocent—or unfeeling—that he or she has nothing to feel guilty about. Some of the things that cause guilt are minor, silly, and frequently more of a problem to us than the other person. Like feeling bad about forgetting the birthday of a second cousin. Sure that's small and insignificant, but people can build up guilt feelings out of very, very little.

Take Jenny A., for example. She constantly felt guilty because she didn't answer letters. Correspondence piled up on her desk, and she just couldn't get down to answering it. Instead of forgetting about it for a while, or just simply forcing herself to do it, she baked a cake, made cookies, etc., whenever she thought about her unanswered correspondence. Which just made her feel even more guilty—and now over something other than her uncompleted tasks.

Sound silly also? Well, the things most people feel guilty about often seem very minor to another person. More to the point, though, once Jenny was able to recognize the circle—guilt leads to eating leads to guilt—she did a complete turnaround. She stopped the cycle of guilty by *doing* what she had long been avoiding, and I don't mean eating. Even more important, by using the Stay Thin method of dealing with guilt—awareness of the situation and control over it rather than mindless eating in response to some vague negative feeling—she lost her weight and kept it off.

There are many constructive ways of fighting old devil guilt, as well as unhappiness, anxiety, frustration, and so on. Physical ways, like jogging or working out in the gym. Mental ways, like reading or taking an adult education course. Emotional ways, like spending more time developing friendships and doing things that make you feel proud of your accomplishments instead of ashamed of your inertia. Even petty, grubby household chores like putting up new shelf paper or darning socks can sometimes be an antidote to gnawing guilt and other negative emotions. In fact, doing *anything*—but eating—is usually helpful.

Ask yourself, "What in my life do I feel guilty about?" Make a list and include *everything*. Be as honest as you can. You're the only one who's going to see this list anyway. Now look it over: which items are based on real causes for guilt, and which ones are simply silly and easily remedied?

Sometimes, as soon as they're out in the open, the reasons for feeling guilty seem ridiculous. Therese M. turned herself into a blimp because she couldn't fulfill her immigrant father's unrealistic scholastic hopes for her. Now she realizes that she did her best and is happy with herself, the only person she has to please anyway. He is the one who, eaten up by disappointment, has the problem.

Unfortunately, for others realization doesn't come that easily or readily. Sam A. also had father problems; his father, sick and old, languished in a distant nursing home. Sam found it emotionally difficult, and physically close to impossible to visit him often. Somehow, his eating binges coincided with the weekends when he felt he should be visiting his ailing father.

Confronted with this fact by his wife, Sam could not just snap his fingers and make the problem disappear. But he is thinking about it, and finally becoming aware of his problem. Soon he'll start considering possible solutions, such as writing his father long, chatty letters, sending little gifts, visiting once a month, and making sure he keeps very occupied on the weekends so that when "Saturday afternoon fever" strikes, he's better able to resist it without bingeing.

As Sam learned, if you're feeling guilty, overeating is one of the finest methods of self-punishment yet devised. It stands shoulder to shoulder with alcoholism as a way of getting back at yourself without being aware of what you're doing. If you feel guilty and you punish yourself, you don't have to feel guilty any more, do you?

Anger at others, and at yourself, is also a very strong motive for overeating. It's good for:

Anger at your parents. (Feel guilty about not

121

pleasing them, and in some cases, not even liking them? Overeat, turn yourself into a person who physically repels them. It's a great way to shunt the guilt of not loving on to them.)

Anger at your friends. (You've decided that they're not supportive enough and often not even there enough when you need them? Then turn to food for friendship; it's a readily available companion in our society.)

Getting back at your spouse. (He or she sometimes infuriates you or disappoints you? Well, food doesn't. Now's your chance.)

Such self-destructive behavior will "work" in the short run whenever you want feelings of guilt or anger to evaporate. And not just in regard to yourself, your parents, your friends, or your spouse, but anyone who hasn't treated you right, or vice versa. But the cycle is self-perpetuating: you eat because you feel guilty and/or angry; and you feel guilty and angry for having eaten. Which makes you feel even worse. Need I say more?

Another emotion that is never helpful and causes some of the worst kinds of unhappiness is self-pity. It's a waste of feeling and energy in any situation, but it is especially destructive when combined with attempts to lose weight and keep it off. For example, self-pity that you have to watch your weight; self-pity that you can't eat and drink whatever and whenever you want; self-pity that you have to deny yourself, say no to yourself, punish yourself with abstinence.

The trouble with self-pity is that it leads to even

more eating and drinking for solace. And if you do that, you'll *really* have something to feel sorry for yourself about. While you can make some of the other negative emotions work for you, self-pity very seldom leads to positive action.

So the minute you start feeling sorry for yourself, work to pull out of it. Sometimes it helps to talk to a friend who is rather tough-minded—one who won't join you in your wallowing but will kindly but firmly advise you to get off your butt and do something about the problem. Call *this* friend instead of the Bleeding Heart who will cry along with you.

Or find a cure yourself. Think about something that has nothing to do with food—something to do, something to read, something to wear, whatever. Michele H. has a habit which she swears pulls her out of the self-pity blahs. Whenever she is feeling sorry for herself, she turns on the TV and watches soap operas. Those people have such awful problems, they never seem to solve them, and they all seem to be mopey, weepy, and miserable all the time," Michele notes. "It makes me so impatient with them that I jump up, turn off the TV, and get mad at them. By that time, I've completely forgotten my own troubles."

Loneliness. Frustration. Boredom. Depression. Anxiety. It's very likely that you have often turned to food in response to these emotions because you can't handle them. But everyone has these feelings at times, and not everyone overeats.

Although in our society, everyone's always supposed to be "up," there's nothing shameful, for example, about occasionally feeling bored or lonely. In fact, there are times of the year when it's almost epidemic. Many people feel loneliest at Christmas and New Year's. Many are bored on Sunday, when there's no work, the stores aren't open, and "everyone else" is off doing something with their friends, lovers, or families.

Most people find it hard to admit to loneliness or boredom, though, as if there were some stigma attached to them, even though everyone else feels these emotions too. It's perfectly natural. Take a look at boredom—which commonly leads to overeating. You operate at a certain high level all day. After work comes a period when you don't have to achieve, you don't have to compete, you don't have to bother to express yourself aggressively. It's boring for many. You've had your motor running all day; now you're idling. And like many people in that predicament, you eat.

But while everyone has various stresses and strains, and experiences one or another kind of unhappiness, or even all kinds, not everyone responds to them the way you do. Most thin people don't feed their faces when they're bored, anxious, lonely, or depressed. They've found better outlets. Those are the people who are interested in so many things that, no matter how much spare time they have, they can always fill it up. They are the ones with hobbies, sports, and exercises that they enjoy, or perhaps the ones who simply like to sit alone and think or work. Why not learn a lesson from them? Next time you have a few minutes to spare, or are bored, ask yourself what things you'd really like to do if you could get up the momentum. Sometimes, boredom is simply a case of inertia, and can be cured by a little imagination.

Also, be careful not to let the person who constantly eats to cope with his stresses and crises and never gains an ounce get you so down that it drives you to overeating in envy and despair. We all know someone who just never seems to gain weight, just as we all know someone who never has a cavity, or who can read the phone book without glasses at the age of sixty-five, or who can smoke three cigarettes a day and never get hooked beyond that. There's only one way to cope with those types: laugh it off, forget it, chalk it up to luck, and don't try to emulate them. Most of us aren't so lucky. If we sin, we pay—in pounds.

Finally, it is not only emotions that lead to inappropriate food drives which in turn lead to bingeing. Some people have certain times of the day, or days of the week, or even seasons of the year when the bingeing urge seems particularly hard to resist.

Many women find that their eating habits fluctuate according to their menstrual cycle. "Don't talk to me about premenstrual tension," Helen C. exploded. "I don't seem to get the usual symptoms, like headaches, cramps or a bloated feeling. I just get cravings—like a pregnant woman. I've learned to watch out at that time and keep a tight rein on myself, but it seems unfair to have to go through this struggle every month." What helps her now is that she's aware of her problems, and is prepared to deal with it in advance, albeit, in more ways than one, with clenched teeth.

Henry Q. finds that it's winter that is most difficult for him. "I'm so damned cold all the time. I eat just to keep warm. Honest. I know it doesn't work, but I can't seem to stop. In the summer, the problem just vanishes." People who feel the heat keenly, and mind it, may have the opposite response: warm weather triggers their cravings for long (sweet) cool drinks, frozen desserts, ice cream—anything that gives the illusion of relief from the heat.

These are some of the traps Mother Nature keeps baited for you. Learn to recognize them, and start a campaign to overcome your particular tough time. The focus here must be on the word "recognize"; if you're aware of your patterns of weakness and vulnerability, you'll be able to take hold and do something about it. Before it's too late.

But you also have to recognize that you're eating and what you're eating. This would seem obvious to those with normal eating habits, but bingers know better. "It's mindless," admitted Jay M. "I hardly know what I'm doing when a binge strikes. I couldn't tell you later precisely what I had—or even whether it was good or bad."

Awareness of what's leading to the binge, and consciousness of what you're doing during it, is the only possible key to ending it.

I've given you a lot of examples of the types of problems and unhappinesses that lead to bingeing because hopefully, you will have recognized your own problem in at least one of those cases.

Step one in thwarting any of these unhappy emotions or situations is to recognize what is going on. You must work to uncover the source of those feelings that are troubling you and leading you to binge. The next time you are about to "go crazy" or out of control, you must stop and try to understand what you're really feeling—which isn't hunger. What is causing this sudden food craving tonight? What was I thinking about when I started to think about food? What has been troubling me? That kind of awareness is the halfway mark—at least—on the road to solving your problems, and not just your bingeing ones by the way.

It also helps to think back to the times in the past when you binged. Usually there's a certain pattern, although you may never have realized it. What emotions tended to set you off? Or what problems tended to provoke your responses? If you "go crazy" as George R. used to, what made you go temporarily insane? George was able to pinpoint the feeling—his frustration about his job. Sam was able to pinpoint the feeling—his guilt about his elderly father. And Terry finally learned that stuffing up his emotions when his wife left led to stuffing up his face.

Believe it or not, making the connection between feelings and food is one of the hardest parts of successfully Staying Thin. Even accepting the fact that such a connection exists is difficult for many people. Most of us try to convince ourselves that our weight is physiologically predetermined in some way. We tell ourselves fibs: that we eat like pigs because we're incredibly hungry; or because something is wrong with our metabolism; or that something external "just comes over us." Somehow these excuses make overeating more respectable, as if it was some sort of an exotic, incurable disease.

But overeating in most cases has more of a psychological than a physiological cause. Think of all those times you binged at midnight, after eating a perfectly fine dinner at seven o'clock. Or you had half a chocolate cake after eating a quarter of a pound of cookies. It wasn't your body but your mind that was compelling you to behave in such a strange and self-destructive way. And as a result, only your mind—not your body—can straighten you out. If you don't give some thought as to what is causing this behavior, you are doomed to repeat it again and again.

It also helps to realize that there's nothing wrong with feeling some of the emotions that lead you to binge. Like loneliness at Christmas, and occasional anger at friends, everyone is prey to such responses. This is an important realization because it helps you dispel any feelings of guilt you may have over these feelings you can't control.

The most important step for you to take though is to concentrate on making that all-important distinction between psychological craving and physical hunger every time you think about responding to an irrational eating impulse.

From now on, every single time (and even if you slip, you must do it the next time), you are thinking of eating when you shouldn't, you must stop (if you can), and ask yourself some very pertinent questions:

Am I really hungry?

When did I eat last?

Am I anxious about something?

Would eating help solve that?

Is there some specific problem bothering me?

Would eating solve that problem?

Am I feeling guilty, frustrated, whatever?

Why?

Would eating change that?

The last time I felt this way, and went ahead and binged, did eating solve anything?

Your next step (which we'll discuss in more detail in future chapters) is to find a new and better way to handle these negative feelings of guilt, inadequacy, resentment, unhappiness, etc. Handling these feelings is the crucial step. Having realized that you became overweight because you made the wrong response, that is, you responded to your emotions or external circumstances rather than to a physical need for food (probably behavior learned as a child), you must now learn to make the right response as an adult. And remember that there's nothing bad about having these negative emotions, because it's not the emotions but your *response* to them that's wrong. And Staying Thin is a matter of finding the right response.

You're not bad or even weak because you overate when you shouldn't have. Think of how strong you are to have been able to reduce all those times. Think of the will power you *have* exercised. Focus on the times you *stopped* yourself from bingeing. Your problem has simply been that you went about trying to solve your problem or fight your emotions in the wrong way.

Awareness is the beginning of moving beyond the control of outside forces, a way to begin mastering, instead of being manipulated by people, by life, by candy bars. When you succeed in this, not only will you be prepared to fight back when the next onslaught comes, but you will gain confidence that you can fight—and that you can *win*. And that confidence will spill over into every part of your daily existence. Your job. Your social circle. Your love life.

The benefits of self-awareness and self-control are many more than just Staying Thin.

8
Finding
the
Right Response

Being in control is a high in itself. Knowing *why* you're mindlessly reaching for food, as you should have begun to understand from the preceding chapter, is a crucial step toward controlling that behavior in the future.

Indeed, you may not only become aware now of your *own* overeating patterns, but you may start noticing other people's wrong or compulsive eating habits as well. Maybe there's a woman in the office next to yours who routinely, automatically, buys a Danish to eat with her morning coffee. Maybe your best friend reaches for a caramel every time he or she has to make a difficult phone call. Or maybe your husband or wife dips his or her hand in and out of the peanuts while reading the evening paper. (Hey—what are

131

those peanuts doing there in the first place?)

Now that you've analyzed the emotional patterns that have led you to mindlessly overeat in the past, you no longer have to behave like a rat being guided (or rather misguided) in a laboratory. You are a free human being, with the power to direct your life. Maybe you learned to overeat during a difficult search for love, or as a response to unhappiness, or to other problems. But now that you know what you're doing, you can start to unlearn that behavior and choose a better route.

Remember that this is not only true for overeating. Maybe you've been living mindlessly in other self-destructive ways as well, perhaps smoking or drinking too much. You are not more doomed to stay that way than you are to have a chronic weight problem. But it's usually best to work on only one crutch at a time. After you've built up your confidence by Staying Thin for a while, you can then most effectively turn to those problems—using the same principles as you've learned here: awareness and control.

As for Staying Thin, the last chapter was the time to look into yourself and find out what problems and emotions were leading you to make the wrong responses to replace them, thereby paving the way for positive change.

To figure out the right response for you, that is, a nonfood response to go to whenever your tail is being pinched (because hopefully you're no longer going to indulge at those times now that you understand the mechanism that makes you overeat), it is necessary for you to make a list of the things you really enjoy doing (other than eating and cooking, of course).

Some people get bogged down temporarily because they can only think of the "big" pleasure packages in life, like skiing or playing a set of tennis doubles. And as a patient in one class aptly pointed out, "I can't go to Aspen every time I'm trying to fight the urge to have a chocolate chip cookie." That's true, but there are also many small pleasures in life that can dissipate that sudden, violent "Big Mac attack."

The kinds of activities that work as substitutes for eating are totally different for you, for a math professor, for a gardener, for a trial lawyer, or for a bus driver. Athletic, hyperactive types find relief in exercise, competition, motion; reflective types are comforted by words—reading or writing may work best for them. Artistically inclined people may like to design and execute craft projects, redecorate rooms, visit museums. Very sociable, outgoing people like to chat, meet friends, talk on the phone, and plan parties. And some people so love their work that they would consider an extra hour at the office to finish up their projects a treat. To a mathematician, a new theorem might constitute pure bliss; to a new mother, a trip to the zoo with her child might be a peak experience.

Be sure that you're not including on your list activities that you think you should like (reading Proust, going to a physics lecture). Do only what you really enjoy. If you're a sedentary type and stuck on soap operas, or long to curl up under the electric blanket for an afternoon nap, *do* it if you can. Love to spend money on books, gadgets, funny greeting cards or blown-glass lizards? Indulge. Remember, your object is to find substitutes that are not fattening. Beyond that, anything goes. Even daydreaming is just fine, if that's your thing, and if it's not about food.

So include in your list all of the nonfood activities that give you even a modicum of pleasure and could therefore serve as a reasonable substitute—or at least a short-term diversion—for what you shouldn't be doing, namely eating. Manicuring (or pedicuring) your nails, writing a note to your college roommate, phoning a pal to arrange a dinner, or gossip over another friend, shopping for fabric to make new clothes, walking the dog, going to the P.O. for stamps, etc. To some of you these may seem like chores, but they're included because many people derive pleasure from minor accomplishments.

Don't be afraid to list something that may seem small and silly to you. Elaine L., a secretary, admits that she likes to get up from her desk every few hours, walk to the ladies' room and put on some fresh perfume. The slight physical activity uses up some of her nervous energy. She likes to sniff the fresh perfume. And the glimpse of her slimming figure in the mirror reminds her of her goal to stay a thinner, more attractive woman.

Tom R., a writer who works at home, overcomes the lure of his all-too-accessible kitchen by taking a break from time to time to listen to a few minutes of a favorite record. He says that he tries to anticipate the almost claustrophobic feeling that

134

"I've got to eat or explode" by taking the break *before* his tension builds too high.

Eileen W., another patient, made a list that read as follows:

Drink herbal tea.

Schedule something for myself over the week-end, like a museum or a play.

Think about it.

Look forward to it.

Take a bubble bath.

Hook rugs.

Buy myself something special like flowers or a scarf.

Note that Eileen lists not one, but a variety of activities, and different types of activities as well. This makes her response more likely to be successful than Elaine's, who may get tired of hers, or be forced to abandon it by colleagues blasted out of the office by an excess of perfume. The clue to success is to have a variety of responses, to vary them, and to keep adding new ones. This list shouldn't be static: add more next month; take those that didn't work for you away.

Sam made his list over a period of a week, by writing down each night which of his minor activities during that day he had found relaxing, distracting and enjoyable.

Take a hot shower.

Go through next week's *TV Guide*.

Read *Time* magazine.

Watch Johnny Carson.

Play a show tune on the piano.

Pat the dog.

Walk the dog.

Go through the mail.

Throw old magazines away.

Read *Playboy*.

Call Janet.

Make a self-improvement list (another one!).

Read the classified ads in the back of the newspaper.

Plan an imaginary vacation.

Balance the checkbook.

Daydream about what it would be like to be rich (and have a checkbook that always balances).

Now, none of these is earth-shattering, but any one of them can occupy and please him long enough to keep him from reaching for food when those "bad vibes" hit. So for this patient, they did the trick.

Furthermore, Sam did some manipulating of his list that made the right response work more often for him. He realized that some things on his list could be done every day (take a shower, walk the dog, etc.), others could be done only once a week (call Janet, whom he was now friends with but no longer dating, and so really couldn't call her every day, read *Time* magazine, etc.), and some were monthly (read *Playboy,* balance checkbook).

So once he became aware of this distribution, he began to space his tasks out so he would always have something to turn to. Even though *TV Guide* and *Time* both came out on Mondays, he started buying them on separate days—and on days when he wasn't going to call Janet. Even within the day, he began spacing out tasks so he would have something he would enjoy doing whenever he thought he would really prefer food. For example, he began to save reading the mail for when he needed to divert himself from overeating; he had a video-tape machine and began recording the Carson show to watch the next day when he needed to distract himself, etc.

Does this give you some ideas about how to best handle your list?

Eventually Sam's (and your) list may include things he should do as well as things he likes to do: "Call Aunt Jane in the nursing home," "get the car inspected," "take the dog to the vet," and other necessary chores. These also serve as substitutes for sinful snacking. But in the beginning, some people find the avoidance of food so punishing that it's best not to substitute anything for eating that isn't pure pleasure or amusement.

For now, keep the right responses positive. Things that you like to do. Things you can look forward to. In the very beginning, you may even indulge yourself a little more: once in a while take a little longer with a pleasant long-distance phone call; use a classier brand of bubble bath; take the dog for a manicure. The right response—your substitute for bingeing on food—is your own best reward.

When you choose to do these substitute activities is also important. Don't wait until you have a half a chocolate cake in front of you to pick up your favorite magazine. If you know ahead of time that at certain hours, or when certain feelings strike, they trigger your vulnerability to food, you can protect yourself by preparing in advance to start these activities. Sam found midnight the most difficult time, for example, so he saved his favorite daily task (reading the mail) for then.

In order to make the response work, however, it must be the right response for you—not Sam, or Elaine, or your spouse, or your friend. Watching a sports game on television may be all it takes to turn your mind away from food, while another person may find sports so dull and irritating that it drives him or her straight to the icebox. Phoning a friend, reading a good book, or writing a page in a diary may be super therapy for some people, while it may drive others up the wall. A brisk walk or a fast game of tennis or handball does the trick best for some, while others find that a twenty-minute catnap, à la Winston Churchill, refreshes them and tones down their food cravings along with the accumulated stress of the day.

Also where you conduct your right response is as important as what your response is. Go over your list and see how many of those favorite things you've gotten in the habit of doing in the kitchen (reading the mail, watching a TV program if you have a set in there, etc.). *Then change rooms.* Never do any of your right responses in the kitchen or you'll soon turn to the wrong responses again.

Actually, it's a good idea, when possible, to place these substitutes for food somewhere on the way to the kitchen. Thus, Jan no longer reads *Esquire*—her favorite magazine—in the kitchen while she's eating. Instead, she puts it on the side of the dining room table, on the way to the kitchen. Then, when the pangs strike, and she walks toward the kitchen, she stops to read an *Esquire* article instead of going in the wrong room to do the wrong thing.

You may find it helpful to set up a special, non-food, "enjoyment" area between your most frequented space and the kitchen. That book you've been wanting to get into, your knitting, even your barbells, the crossword puzzle, etc., should all go there. Fight pleasure with pleasure.

If the "joy of eating" is to be taken away from a dieter, at least for a while, it must be replaced with another joy, or the dieting and Staying Thin attempts will fail. Some choose the joy of sex as a good substitute. Or the joy of work—as long as it doesn't get to be as obsessive and self-destructive a habit as eating. A little exercising. Now that's a good idea.

Only you will know what works best to stop you in your relentless and inexorable march to the kitchen. You won't have to do this forever. But at the beginning, simple adherence to the daily diet is usually not enough to deter you consistently from the dirty deed—the binge. For now, you have to substitute something positive for the desirable food. After you've gained confidence that you don't have to eat every time the craving hits, after you understand each time why the craving hits, and as a result keep your weight down for a long time, Staying Thin will be its own reward.

STOPPING THE WRONG RESPONSE

It would be great if every time you were about to binge, you stopped, realized that you were responding to an emotion rather than to real hunger, and decided either not to give in to it or, as we've just discussed, to dissipate those cravings with alternative activities.

Yes, it *would* be great, like world peace, an end

140

to famine, and other things that will never happen. It's highly unlikely that you'll be able to avoid binges 100 percent, at least at the beginning of your new program for Staying Thin permanently.

Therefore, the next step is for you to learn how to stop yourself from making the wrong response if it happens, and before you end up in Fat City. Now maybe you think that once that urge hits you, you simply can't stop yourself, even if you realize both what you're doing and what's causing it to occur. But you can if you understand that overeating doesn't just "happen." Eating, like everything else, is a series of acts that can be stopped at any point along the way, once you're aware of what's involved and make attempts to control it.

For example, May D. was fifty-five pounds overweight before her last diet. Every night she watched television from nine until eleven, religiously. She brooked no interruptions; if the phone rang, she asked the person to call back. If a neighbor dropped by, she wouldn't talk to them until the program was over.

There was something else that she always did just as faithfully. After the first hour of watching the tube, she invariably got a craving for something to munch on. So she would always stroll to the refrigerator for a snack before the ten o'clock show would go on.

Now let's analyze what really was taking place here. The TV program ended. The first commercial appeared. This served as a cue to leave her seat and start moving in the direction of the kitchen. Obviously, if she had never left her seat in the first place, she would never have landed in the kitchen. But try to convince May not to get up! After all, she had done it this way every night for several years (except during a blackout, when she stayed in the kitchen altogether). The ten o'clock kitchen break had become as ingrained a habit as brushing her teeth, locking the front door at night, or brewing a fresh pot of coffee in the morning.

Of course May would be best off striking out the first step in the chain—in this case, getting up from the chair when the commercial comes on. But even if she failed to stop an undesirable chain of behavior at the first step, she could try to strike out any of the subsequent steps along the way. Although she didn't realize it until later, she wasn't lost the minute she got up from the chair. She wasn't lost until she swallowed the first bite. (There are some people who can stop themselves after one bite, but they're so rare that it's hardly even worth mentioning them.) May could also walk in a different direction, to the bathroom, perhaps, or out onto the terrace to look at the stars. But to her, that walk to the kitchen was as inevitable as the pounds it put on her.

Now, she could have put up roadblocks (as we discussed) to divert her interest and energy on the way to the kitchen. But for her, that walk into the kitchen was like one all-consuming act and she wouldn't have noticed anything along the way, because she was only thinking of the final step in her chain of behavior.

We'll discuss later actual stoppers she could have put in the kitchen, such as a full-length mirror, a photograph on the refrigerator, wrapped foods, etc. These are all deterrents, attempts to jar her so that she could stop her self-destructive behavior en route.

But in addition to the physical roadblocks, she could also set up psychological ones. Instead of continuing to make her nightly forays in a completely mechanical manner, she could become *aware* of all the steps involved in her snacking and try to break one link in the chain somewhere along the way—the earlier in the sequence the better. It's easier to stop one little act than an automatic cycle.

So let's look at what really happens whenever May—and perhaps you—succumbs to that urge for a nightly binge.

1. The program goes off.

2. The commercial goes on.

3. May gets up.

4. She walks across the living room.

5. She goes through the foyer.

6. She passes the dining alcove.

7. She enters the kitchen.

8. She walks over to the refrigerator.

9. She puts her hand on the door.

10. She presses the lever.

11. The door opens.

12. She looks around.

13. She spies a piece of cake.

14. She takes a plate out of the cupboard.

15. She puts the cake on it.

16. She takes a fork out of the drawer.

17. She takes a napkin out of the cupboard.

18. She carries the fork, napkin, and the plate out of the kitchen.

19. She passes the dining alcove.

20. She goes through the foyer.

21. She walks across the living room.

22. She sits down.

23. She picks up her fork.

24. She cuts a piece of cake.

25. She lifts it to her lips.

26. She eats it.

Now, there were twenty-six separate steps required in order for May to have her snack. It didn't "just happen" as she always assumed. Even if she couldn't break the chain at the beginning, she had twenty-five other opportunities to do so.

If *any one* of her responses had been stopped along the way, May would never have eaten the cake, the pie, or whatever her refrigerator held in store.

Obviously, the best place to stop an undesirable chain of behavior is right at the beginning. A number of psychological studies have been done in this area which prove that the point at which it's hardest to break the chain is when you're nearest your goal; the closer you get to the cake, the harder it is not to eat it. But that doesn't mean May *can't* do it at the end; only that it's much easier to stop the chain of behavior somewhere in the first twenty-five steps. (In fact, during the first twelve would be the easiest—before she was even tempted by looking at the food.)

Think of how your own chain of behavior results in self-indulgence. Maybe it's passing a neighborhood pastry shop. Or getting out of bed at midnight to binge. Make a mental (or actual) note of *all* the different steps involved in your final negative behavior. Try to be aware of these steps the next time ou go through them. Try to break the chain *at every single step*. Sure it's hard to overcome a completely automatic activity. But it's not that difficult to stop one of twenty-five small pieces of behavior along the way.

So stop focusing only on the final act (eating), and think throughout of what you're doing to get to it. It's never too late to stop a negative chain of behavior—until you've actually swallowed the food.

CHANGING TO THE RIGHT THOUGHTS

There are more ways to keep yourself from making the wrong response than just by physically stopping yourself in the midst of a chain of events. One can also stop a negative chain of thought by substituting a positive one for it that leads to food as inevitably as the physical chain does. Sometimes this is a bit harder because while no one can be eating every minute of their waking day, some compulsive overeaters are thinking about food both consciously and subliminally almost as often.

The person with a constant weight problem is often obsessed with food. He thinks about it more than he does anything else. (Indeed, for many, that is the real national pastime.) How many times a day do thoughts like these grip your mind:

I'll never be able to stay thin.

I'm hungry again. This isn't fair.

One little cookie won't make any difference.

I wonder how a pizza would taste right now.

It isn't worth the torture. Why not just give up and be fat and happy?

One hamburger won't hurt.

Hamburgers are pure protein.

As often as you do this consciously, there are times that you do it without really realizing it. Day after day, you engage in a lot of thinking, much of which you're barely aware of. If you're going on a vacation, a picture of a beach may occasionally pop to mind beforehand. If you're inviting people to your house, a fleeting image of the forthcoming event may cross your mind as you're shopping, cleaning, cooking, etc. If your child's teacher sends a note home asking to see you in conference, you may try to put it out of your mind, but "what ifs" keep popping up.

You're thinking almost all the time, even when you're sleeping. Researchers have found that everyone, even those who swear they never dream, engage in about one and a half hours of dreaming at night—every night. So the mind is an instrument that never sleeps.

But when it comes to food, large numbers of people, overweight people, or about forty to eighty million Americans (depending on which statistics you believe) use this amazing instrument in the wrong way. You think about the delicious cheesecake in the refrigerator, the lasagna in the oven, the ice-cold bottle of beer to be had. You're often thinking of food, even though you may not always be aware of these thoughts. No wonder in the past it's been hard for you to Stay Thin.

Most of these thoughts can drive you right to the fathouse. But there are ways to control, override, or disperse obsessive food thoughts, which have been frequently and successfully used by behavior therapists with food-obsessive patients. Some of these we've already discussed, but here are a few others as well which you can use to stop yourself when you're about to make the wrong response.

USING PRINCIPLES OF ALCOHOLICS ANONYMOUS FOR FOOD

Most of life's problems are best handled by minimizing them, e.g., "My mother-in-law will be here for ten days and I've got to stop thinking about it and making such a big deal over it. I'll just have as little do with her as possible once she arrives."

Or if you haven't been to the dentist for three years, worrying about it for two weeks beforehand, and imagining all the things that could possibly be wrong with your mouth, is just going to make you more apprehensive and accomplish nothing. It's better to try to forget about it, and when you do think of it, convince yourself that a little cleaning is all that will be necessary.

There's a mother-in-law, dentist or occasional

thorn-in-the-flesh in everyone's life, and usually it's best with those things to try not to make a big deal out of it. But there's one problem that's best handled not by minimizing the situation or consequences but by maximizing it: Eating what you shouldn't.

It isn't going to do you any good to tell yourself that "it's just a little piece of cake. How can that possibly matter?" It *does* do you good—especially at the moment you're trying to stop yourself from having it—to say to yourself, "That one little piece of chocolate has 150 calories. Two of them (which I'll no doubt have after the first, at least) have 300 calories. That's practically the equivalent of a whole nutritious meal."

Actually, it may be the equivalent of more than a meal, because most people, if they can't resist the first two pieces, may not be able to resist the fourth plus, either. As it's sometimes said, "A sliver leads to a slice leads to a slab leads to a slob." All it takes to get a foodaholic started again is that one little piece of chocolate cake, just as all it takes to get the alcoholic started again is just one little drink. Most can't stop once they get started, and neither can most foodaholics.

Borrow AA's principle that one drink is to die. Sure, that's pretty dramatic. But if you think of how obesity can kill, it may be more true than you'd like to believe. One little drink isn't going to kill anyone either. But if an alcoholic has one drink, he's likely to have ten. Remind yourself that all you have to do to fall off your program is to have that one compulsive little bite. And convince yourself before you start that it's the beginning of the end.

ONE DAY AT A TIME

Now, let's borrow another AA principle (since it's a group that's had outstanding success with a different type of compulsive behavior) to concentrate only on today and handle weight loss one day at a time. Losing weight, if done this way, is not an impossible task. Remember that's the way you made yourself fat—one day at a time—and it's also the way you can make yourself thin again.

Don't let the notion of "forever" scare you. There are days when it seems so disheartening; when life without ever having another piece of mocha-fudge layer cake hardly seems worth it to some; when a birthday without a birthday cake just seems so meaningless.

When you get into one of *those* moods, and are about to use it to justify eating something you shouldn't, stop yourself by refusing to think about what will happen in the future. Forget about tomorrow. Just say to yourself, *"Today* I will attend this wedding and will not overeat. I'll worry about what I'm going to do tomorrow when it gets here." Or, "Today I will turn down my mother's apple pie. I'll decide tomorrow how to handle tomorrow's temptations."

Arlene J. attributes this attitude to keeping her thin for three years now. "One week after I had finally reached 109 pounds, my goal-weight of a lifetime, I found myself at a restaurant on a first date with a man I had liked for a long time," she recalls. "Everything was going beautifully when he asked me what I wanted for dessert. I was a little stoned, and bad thoughts can really grab hold of you then. And it hit me like a brick that the diet I would be on for the rest of my life would never allow me any gooey desserts.

"Well, my sense of loss was so deep, I felt as if my best friend had died. I started shaking, and tears were filling my eyes. I just wanted that dessert so badly.

"And then I realized that I could always go off my diet tomorrow," she added. "No one was forcing me to stay thin. But for that night, I was going to turn down the offer for that dessert."

You can do what Arlene did whenever temptation seems too much for you. Say things like:

For now I'm going to pass up this pizza. (God knows what I'll do tomorrow.)

Right now, I do not want bread. (I'll reconsider that decision tomorrow.)

I'm going to be strong today and pass this candy bar up. (If I feel weak tomorrow, I might have one.)

If you can just get through your todays without overeating, you'll never have to worry about your tomorrows.

WORK TO CHANGE NEGATIVE THINKING

It also helps in handling the mood for food to think in terms of change rather than denial. One of the most difficult things to accept once you get thin is that there are certain foods that you will never eat again (or will eat only in negligible quantities)

151

as Arlene sadly came to realize in the restaurant that night.

Now, the thought that you will lose a dear food friend blows many people's minds to such a degree that they promptly devour an entire box of donuts, a half a pizza, or whatever it was that they were not supposed to eat again, in order to comfort themselves over their loss.

But a better way is to stop focusing on the foods you aren't going to have, and stop using words you've come to associate with deprivation. Instead, think of what you can have, and say that to yourself in a positive way.

The unaware people trying to Stay Thin say things to themselves like:

"I'll never again have a whole pizza."

"I don't dare touch cake any more."

"I've got to stay away from ice cream."

"I am off candy bars now."

Rather than focusing on avoiding certain foods, think in terms of indulging in others. Your new regimen no doubt includes lots of vegetables, salads, proteins, etc. So get in the habit of saying (and thinking) things like:

"I'm going to switch to lots of vegetables."

"I can have all the salad I want."

"I'm going to exchange ice cream cones for low calorie drinks."

"I'm going to trade donuts for eggs in the morning."

Think in up terms. You have simply switched some of the foods which you used to eat for others which are better for you, and which you will ultimately learn to like more.

AVOIDANCE

There are a few food situations in which, unfortunately, the only way to stop the wrong response is to avoid the temptation in the first place.

For example, if you burn severely every time you go to the beach, the most obvious way to forestall this pain is to take your vacation in the mountains, or in some other location where you will not be exposed to strong sun, no matter how much you like to sunbathe.

You have to do the same with food in some situations until Staying Thin becomes a part of your life. One patient described how every time she shopped at her favorite department store, she passed by a bakery shop two doors away. The delicious odors and sights invariably led to entering the shop and not infrequently to making a little purchase (often on the pretext of bringing home a treat for the children) which then paved the road to an unanticipated binge.

Her solution to the problem was not to shop at all (she was desperate), but I suggested something much simpler: that she approach the department store from another direction. "Oh but that would mean walking an entire extra block," she replied.

"What's wrong with that?" I asked.

"It takes time."

When I pointed out to her how much time she was spending bingeing as a result of her purchase (not to mention worrying about it before and afterwards), she saw how simple the solution to her problem really was.

The avoidance strategy is recommended for those problem behaviors that occur time after time in the same situation and which *can* be avoided, like the bakery shop on the way to the department store, or a pizza stand in a multientranced subway. Unfortunately, avoidance doesn't work as well for the unpredictable times of temptation when the food is literally thrust in front of you, like the box of chocolates delivered by Western Union, your roommate's wedding reception, or a boring dinner party where there's nothing to do but eat.

Now, it's not true that all you have to do is avoid predictable food temptations and hallelujah, your weight problems will be solved and your scales will miraculously dip. That would be a shortsighted solution. You must learn to face tempting situations repeatedly and not succumb to them. Food doesn't just go away; wherever you turn, it's there.

And, by the way, when you're about to indulge, it's very damaging to say to yourself, "Just this one time," or, "This is the last time." Indeed, never say anything like that to yourself because it isn't true, and it just gives you an excuse to eat four times as much as you would have eaten normally.

The key to the suggestions in this chapter is again *awareness: awareness* that you've got a craving (not a hunger) for food; knowing you must try to find other activities to draw you away from it; breaking down your bingeing behavior and trying

154

to stop it at each step along the way; being *aware* of your food thoughts and then starting to change them so you can benefit from your new attitudes; thinking only of one day at a time, and thinking in terms of change rather than deprivation. And in those few instances in which the situation is just too much for you, gracefully practicing total avoidance rather than permitting yourself to engage in mindless and unaware eating.

And if you handle situations in these ways, the process of Staying Thin will never be biting off more than you can chew.

9
Changing
Your
World

The past few chapters were aimed at helping you to change the way you think as it relates to food. First, understanding that you probably learned to make the wrong response (compulsive overeating) as a child, and that you were most likely taught (and encouraged) to respond in that way by your parents, and perhaps your grandparents.

Next, you learned how these wrong responses have carried over to today, so that whenever you feel anxious, upset, or beset by problems, you still choose the wrong response: eating. Responding correctly (that is, *not* eating as a reaction to various problems and emotions) occurs firstly when you become truly aware of what you're doing, and secondly, when you substitute constructive thoughts or actions for the old self-destructive responses or ideas.

While that will help you handle bingeing, snacking, and general compulsive overeating in the future, there's more to Staying Thin than just fighting the food urge whenever it comes over you. There's also prevention. To Stay Thin permanently, you are going to have to change more than just your reactions to specific situations.

You are going to have to change the world.

Now, don't groan. It isn't as hard as it sounds. Since the world's much too large for us to grasp, we all get through life by paying attention only to specific aspects of it anyway. You don't live in the same physical or psychological world, or see the same things as a Peoria schoolteacher or a South American rancher. You see what's relevant to your space. Furthermore, you're not locked into that world. If you wish, you too can become a Peoria schoolteacher or South African rancher. Or you can simply continue to live where and as you do, but focus on different aspects of your environment. Or focus on the same things—but see them differently.

Fat people, for example, often see Madison Avenue as their enemy. A thin person, watching the same TV program, might ignore or not even notice the food commercials; a fat person would not only be riveted to them but might be personally offended by them. An innocent commercial for Sara Lee is like a rifle trained on their hearts, a bayonet to their growing stomachs. They view the commercial as a direct invitation to them for an offer they know they shouldn't accept. Constant exhortations to buy beauty products may insult fat viewers, because they're useless to them. Why should a woman who is grossly overweight spend hours watching commercials for or reading about hair dyes, makeup, lipsticks, blushers, or fashions that are only going to make her look like a dressed-up elephant? It's like steering a blind woman through a beautiful art gallery and then rubbing in the fact that she can't see the paintings.

Ultimately, many fat people view the world as a place that has no part they can play. They are merely spectators outside a closed door. And inside, the world's treats and pleasures are preempted by and directed toward the enjoyment of thinner folks.

Such a view of the world provides an excellent excuse not even to try to penetrate that barrier. Being blind is an excuse for not enjoying a Rembrandt exhibit. Being overweight is an excuse to sit on the sidelines for all events, except those that pertain to eating.

Even places designed for overweight people are hard for many to stomach. Sally S., an affluent middle-aged tub, felt that even fat farms weren't meant for her. When she went to a $1,000 a week "fat farm"—a present from her husband—she complained afterwards that "all that exercise, dressing up for dinner, massaging, makeup and beauty treatments were lost on me. I felt embarrassed and out of place there." Now if Sally felt out of place *there,* where could she feel comfortable?

But many overweight people see most of the world as a foreign place, an exclusive club they can never join. *Their* world is one in which food predominates: everything is structured around it. They arrange to meet people "for breakfast," "after lunch," and "before dinner"—and as a patient who had once put on 180 pounds admitted, "All day long, I was privately at a meal."

To them, life is a flat plain, marked with soaring pillars of high caloric content. Their daily peak experiences are meals, snacks, and binges. But the normal person's world contains a wide variety of peaks—sports events, movies, friends, hobbies, good books, etc. These are the people who are apt to say, in a busy day, "Oops. I completely forgot to eat lunch today. I got so involved."

Your job, then, is to learn how to fill your landscape with noncaloric joys while diminishing your focus on food.

Think now about the blocks of times when you are most fixated on food. A typical example is right after work, when you're physically tired and mentally exhausted from a demanding day. Studies have shown that there's a definite connection between being tired and overeating, especially since the peppy, active person often doesn't take a break to sit down and eat.

Or perhaps you are most likely to "go bonkers" in midmorning, in an effort to "fuel up" for the day ahead. This is also a typical pattern, exemplified by the person who brings his own breakfast (often his second) to his desk to munch on with his morning coffee.

The danger period probably depends on your schedule, your habits, and even to a small degree, your metabolism. (Although probably less than you would like to believe.) Or it can even be haphazard, which is more difficult to deal with because of the element of unpredictability. Whenever they occur, it's imperative that you fill these periods with some other type of activity.

In order to Stay Thin, you must actively work at focusing your thoughts and actions away from food, which is possible to do if you actively work to direct attention outside of yourself. Now, surrounded by your protective layer of blubber, insulated by excuses, fearful of going out in the world and facing up to all its threats, you probably stay home much more than you should. And at home, there's not much to do. But eat. And so you get fatter, and even more fearful of the world which thinks you look funny. It's a dangerous cycle, and one that's hard to break.

But there is an answer to this. To change, to metamorphose yourself like a caterpillar turning into a butterfly, you must change the world you live in. We'll talk later about changing specific parts of that world—your kitchen, your shopping, your friends. But first, let's discuss how you can change your view of the world and your place in it so you become an insider instead of an outsider.

The secret is to start acting like a thin person. What is there about a thin person's life that's different from yours? Well, the thin person is usually busy, active. "Well of course," I can hear you saying, "because he's thin, he can do all those

160

strenuous, tiring things that I can't do. Of course he's busy and active.''

Did you ever stop to think that maybe you've got it backwards? That maybe he's thin because he's active, not the other way around? While you fill your emptiness with food, what does a thin person do? What does he do with his time? What does he do with his hands? What does he do with his hurt feelings when bad things happen? Eat? Uh-uh.

Take a good long look at the way thin people live. Compare it with the way you live. What does a thin person have that you don't have?

For one thing, probably a membership in the local gym or a tennis club. No matter where you live—big city suburbs, small town, a farm—facilities for exercises are available. Even if such facilities aren't convenient for you, there's always jogging, jumping rope, yoga, calisthenics, and a number of inexpensive equipment-free and healthy forms of exercise that if you really want to, you can even do in the privacy of your own home.

But some people use their weight as an excuse not to exercise, even though it's the best reason for them to do it. When Carla G. was fifty pounds overweight, she admits it was really hard to get herself out on that gym floor with those other women. ''They all looked so thin. Here I was, in an exercise class that was supposed to be for spot-reducing, and I coulnd't see a thing wrong with any of their spots,'' she noted.

''What made me stick with it,'' she went on, ''was realizing that my daughters were ashamed of me, of having a fat mother. They didn't like to bring their friends home after school. And then I noticed that other kids were proud of the way their mothers ran things around the school, you know, the PTA, the Scout troop, the ski club.

"I asked myself why I'd never been tapped for an office, no matter how much scut work I did, and took a hard look at myself. I was dressing as well as I could, but there wasn't much style in the clothes that would fit me. When a person is fat, other people think that they're slobs no matter how neatly they dress."

After a while, Carla found that she actually enjoyed the exercise class which had seemed so boring at first. A camaraderie developed among the class members, some of whom admitted to Carla that they had once been in her situation. These people, rather than despising her because of her weight, as she had feared, were sympathetic and encouraging.

Soon, she went to the class because she enjoyed it, not because she felt guilty about her appearance and its effects on her kids. It didn't happen overnight but ultimately, because she had made friends, lost weight, and improved her figure, she began to feel better about herself. And because she felt better about herself, other people felt better about her. Enough said?

Regular physical activity doesn't mean you have to wake up at seven and exercise until eight. You can exercise by going disco dancing, swimming, skating, or if done brisky, even by walking. In addition there are many built-in ways to exercise and bring more activity into your life without having to go to a gym:

Judy M. had three of the five extension phones in her home removed so that she would have to walk around the house a little more—sometimes even run—in order to answer the phone.

Wanda R., who lived in the upper part of a two-story house in Pelham, tossed out her garbage pails and wastebaskets and bought tiny ones. This forced her to dump her garbage frequently, and to climb up and down the two flights of stairs a few times a day to do so.

And one Wisconsin housewife had another way of forcing herself to expend more energy. "I had the wall to wall carpeting removed and put in a number of small rugs around the house. Then, a couple of times a week, I would take them outside instead of vacuuming them indoors. I'd made a point to really shake those rugs out. I took a belly dancing course once, but I felt I was giving my body even more of a workout with these rugs. I was also glad, at these prices, to save electricity. And I don't care what all the vacuum cleaner commercials say, cleaning your rugs by hand in this manner makes them cleaner than 'the modern way.'"

It's an incontrovertible fact now that regular exercise improves your health across the board. Your heart, your lungs, your digestion, even your skin benefit. But besides being good for your physical health, exercise is good for your mental health too. Indeed, a surprising study recently showed that depressed people derived as much benefit out of running three times a week for fifteen minutes as did a comparable group receiving psychotherapy for the same period of time.

Michael J., a patient who was suffering from mild depression as well as mild overweight, learned this for himself. "After I started running, I almost forgot I was depressed. In fact, I guess I'm not any more," he said.

Michael found the running invigorating, and as he increased the distance he was able to cover, he began to feel very pleased with himself. Now he takes great pride in being a "five-mile-a-day man."

He's lost weight, too, which also makes him proud. Naturally, while he's out running, he isn't eating. Then, at the same time, he's working off excess calories. Finally, the pride he feels at his discipline and accomplishment carries over, so that he just isn't as interested in putting his body down by stuffing it any more.

Some exercise is to be recommended more for its psychological than physical value. Frank H. had always wanted to take up horseback riding, but his parents had been unable to afford riding lessons for him. When he became successful in business, the money didn't matter, but by then he was ashamed to go to the stable because of his weight. "I was afraid the instructor would make some joke about giving the horse a swayback the way my wife did." So Frank began dieting, and managed to shed twenty-five pounds, before indulging in his secret dream.

"The satisfaction of earning a luxury I've

wanted since I was a kid is as much of a high as I get from riding across the fields on a brisk fall day." Frank also works at keeping trim, so he can *keep* riding.

Riding, however, is one of those sports that you can do for hours at a time and never lose weight. Two other kinds of fairly "useless" sports, as far as real weight loss is concerned, are bowling and golf. But for Frank, the joys of riding depended on Staying Thin; they also served to get him out of the house, away from food, and with other people. This worked in the same way as the smaller diversions we discussed in the last chapter: a positive and pleasurable activity to be substituted for eating.

Other "useless" sports are excellent for the same reasons: they open up a new world for you, and help you focus on something besides eating. You also enjoy the sports more if you are thin and lithe, so they give you an incentive to Stay Thin.

Jogging, though not quite as "useless" as some other sports, is really not that helpful as far as burning off calories is concerned. Most people can't or don't run enough to cause any meaningful weight loss. But helping you Stay Thin is another matter. Apparently it's hard to be anxious, depressed, sorry for yourself, or whatever, when you've ventilated all that air through your lungs, pushed all those muscles so far, and had that good swinging sense of being in motion that running provides. Many people have noted an almost mystical "high" that they get when they've been running long distances regularly. A feeling of being "in tune" with life. And if ever anyone needed to feel "in tune," it's someone with a yo-yoing weight problem.

Barbara J., for example, lost her job, broke up with her beau, and had to have extensive dental work—all in a period of three months. "I found it harder and harder to get up in the morning," she remembers now. "I didn't enjoy anything. I was just a low-keyed mess. Everything checked out O.K. physically, so my doctor suggested jogging."

At first it was hard to her to get going, but then "it's a feeling that's almost like euphoria. It got so I wouldn't let anything interfere with my running time. And to think that it doesn't cost me a penny."

But before you decide to run, or ride, or take part in any new activity, learn something about it. There's usually a right way and a wrong way to do anything, whether it's running, riding, or eating. There are plenty of books about running (maybe too many) and indeed, about other sports also. (I recently counted twenty-three currently available just on exercise in one bookstore in Manhattan.) And don't forget to get your doctor's approval if the activity you choose represents a real departure from your usual exercise or nonexercise pattern.

It's important, too, to try to seek out other people interested in the same sports and activities. Running, riding, exercising, etc., can be solitary affairs. But they don't have to be, especially if you join a group or class, or seek others out during breaks. It may also be that you would derive increased benefit from a sport that's more sociable to begin with, like tennis or volleyball. Besides helping you to work off weight and tension, and to fill the vacuum in your life that you've been used to filling with food, these pastimes force you to be with other people.

It's true that for some people, getting (and staying) fat is a way to avoid dealing with others. But deep, deep down, even deeper than this fear of others, there's another feeling that says, "I really do want to be accepted by others. I'm just afraid that they'll reject me, so I reject them first. Or, "I keep myself fat so that I never have 'to be weighed in the balance' (an apt metaphor), 'and found wanting.' " Chances are, if you didn't have that secret longing, you wouldn't periodically put yourself through the torture of dieting, and you wouldn't be working now to Stay Thin, hoping to break a lifelong vicious cycle.

Another thing thin people have that fat people generally don't have is a satisfying hobby—and I don't mean gourmet cooking. Many people enjoy reading or collecting things, but to Stay Thin, what works best is something hand-filling as well as ful-filling. Macramé or woodworking, for example, keeps your hand out of the refrigerator. "Working on a needlework pillow really helps," said Millie. "Just poking the needle in and out of the canvas takes away some of the anger and aggression I feel when I deprive myself of food."

A hobby that's gloriously messy, like working with clay or model airplane glue, can be best of all. No matter how tempting food is to you, it's a pain in the neck to have to put down your work and clean up before eating, especially if you're really getting into what you're doing and plan to go back to it after you eat. Besides which, if your hands are full (and dirty) you probably won't be ferrying food to your mouth.

Adele T., as part of her program to Stay Thin, took a correspondence course in calligraphy. When she got her "diploma," she found that she not only had a new hobby, but a new source of income: the local school asked her to hand-letter all of their diplomas.

"I consider this prize money," Adele says, "like a reward. I never put it into the household kitty, no matter how short I am. I use this money to buy myself things that are rewards for Staying Thin."

Other people have started mail-order businesses, begun teaching Sunday-school classes, taken piano lessons again, and so on. If your mind is full, and your time is taken, you won't be constantly sabotaged by images of forbidden fruit.

Jack R., who had been an overweight recluse, decided to force himself to go out of his house at least two nights a week. But he couldn't just wander around or he'd probably end up walking into a bar or restaurant. So he's studying Spanish at the local adult night school. "It keeps me off the streets," he jokes in Spanish. It also keeps him out of the kitchen.

When Liz S., a rather sedentary (which was her problem) woman, took a course in calculus, her friends thought she was crazy. "What use will you ever have for that?" they all wanted to know. But for Liz, it was something she had always wanted to do because her mind had been lying fallow for years. Now she was getting her mind—instead of her mouth—in gear again.

Like Carla and Frank, Jack and Liz are getting more out of their new activities than a momentary escape from food. While once they were like kids who had nothing to do but get into trouble, now they are enjoying the opportunity to use their minds, fill their hands and their time, and meet people with similar interests. Because they're no longer bored and lonely, they no longer spend so much time thinking about, preparing, and devouring food they don't need. And as they've developed competence, they've developed confidence, which has helped them to Stay Thin, and has had a salutary effect on other areas of their lives as well.

So choose what suits you (and what's available, even if only by correspondence) and make sure it's really fun for you. If not, you will quickly start concentrating on the world of food again.

And don't use money as an excuse for not getting out of the house and doing something to help you focus on new and different things to do. When I suggested a program to Joanne H., she said angrily that "what you are talking about is expensive. Do you know how much it costs to join a gym? And nobody teachers a class for free." What she'd forgotten is that it costs more to be fat.

Besides which, if you can't afford the country club then try the running track at the YMCA or your local high school. School athletic facilities are almost always open to the public at certain hours of each week. Or perhaps there's an inexpensive Y nearby with a swimming pool that you can use for very little.

As for classes and courses, gyms and some college extension courses may be expensive, but here too there's always the Y, and many high schools provide inexpensive adult classes, usually at night. Often there's a wide range of programs; indeed, some offer things like hypnosis and jump-roping (but not together). If the high school in your neighborhood doesn't have what you want, try one in another community. But keep out of their cooking classes.

Sure, eating is one of life's greatest pleasures. But life also has many other pleasures in store for you if you will only seek them out. Your problem has been that you focused too much on the joy of eating and not enough (or at all) on the happiness found in the noncaloric mineral world as opposed to the animal and vegetable one. So join a hiking club. Learn to make jewelry. Actively support a political candidate. Go to the opera.

You can satisfy the natural hunger for pleasure in ways that are enriching rather than self-destructive. Once you change one small part of your environment, you can begin to change your whole life, till it shifts further and further away from a world in which eating was the only activity you ever really enjoyed.

10
Stopping
Snacking

By now you should be filled with plans, armed with lists, and abristle with resolutions to take up new sports, hobbies, and intellectual pursuits so that a whole new (thin!) life opens up for you.

Although these new activities, along with the smaller diversions we also covered earlier, may take up a lot of the time you used to spend eating, there will still be moments, little chinks and crannies of time, that will sneak up on you, and your old desire to snack will return. That ten minutes, for instance, just after you've gotten the family off to school and work, and before you settle down to your morning's schedule; or that twenty-minute break in dinner preparations, when a stiff drink and some cheese and crackers would really hit the spot. Some dieters find that those last moments before bed—while you're locking up and turning out the lights—are the times when temptation is the greatest. And snacking is more than just a little backsliding; it can mean the difference between success and failure in any attempt at weight control.

Eating certain foods is a little like having sex; when you get some, you just want more. And not surprisingly, we've become a nation of snack fiends. The ideal solution would be to break the snacking habit altogether, but for most dieters, that's difficult if not altogether impossible. So the next best thing is to retrain yourself to at least snack properly.

The first and most important step is, once again, to become aware that you *are* snacking. We do it so often that we barely realize it. Few of us adhere strictly to the three-meal-a-day ritual. We are, in fact, a nation of hit-and-run eaters, filling our faces with snacks throughout the day and night. How many times do you take an afternoon break from work by diving into a bag of potato chips? Think of all the hours you sit eating and drinking while glued to the television set. (More on that later.) You mainline daily doses of sweets in the hope of picking up quick energy. You interrupt the tedium of the daily routine by gorging on junk food, or, in some cases, on snacks that are "good for you"—raisins, yogurt, hard cheese— but just as high in calories. In fact, snacking is so much a part of our lives, that we're often unaware of exactly how much we're doing it.

TV snacking is often the worst. In this country, from the time children are very young we encourage the association of TV and eating. We use TV, as we use food, as a kind of pacifier or baby-sitter for when kids get restless. We place children in front of TV sets and then plop their food in front of them. We even refer to frozen meals as TV dinners. Small wonder that when the children grow up, they automatically associate television with food.

For most people, it is a pleasant association. One of the group-patients noted that "eating in front of the television set is more fun than eating at a dining room table, because I don't feel as guilty about it. The room is dark, so it's easy to close my eyes to exactly how much food I'm really consuming."

And snack she does. TV watching is a not-so-tender trap that snares those of us who grew up since the 1940s. That invention led us to become a nation of television watchers. In fact, a recent survey showed that more American families had TV sets than telephones.

Unfortunately, the TV habit has helped to make food junkies out of us. Most American people spend an inordinate amount of their at-home time in front of the television set. Overweight people especially. The nonstop temptations flickering in front of us subliminally—and not so subliminally— are constantly telling us to indulge. Which is just the opposite of the Stay Thin message, or that of any other weight maintenance program for that matter.

And TV food pitches are hard for us to resist. The images that dance across our screens are of delicious food (in glorious color), served in spacious, spotless kitchens that never seem to get cluttered, messy, or smoky. Or else the pictures are of fast foods promising instant gratification—McDonald's burgers, Kentucky Fried Chicken, Sara Lee cake—with no more strenuous effort required to get to them than the tearing off a wrapper or the opening of a carton.

If you are immobile before the set for long stretches of time, you're literally a sitting target for this commercial barrage. Even if you were to somehow remove the commercials, or flee the room while they're on (without wandering into the kitchen), the problem remains. Think of all those scenes in situation comedies in which the family is assembled around a table, eating. Or the entertainment scenes in which they're snacking and drinking. Or the party scenes where they're gorging. And irony of ironies—the people you see eating nonstop in those scenes and in commercials (with the possible exception of those spots for Italian spaghetti sauces, which show pleasingly plump women serving downright fat men) are all thin.

What is particularly damaging about this TV temptation is that often we are not even aware of it. We lose track of our forays to the fridge and make those repeat trips almost automatically. Television often hits us where it hurts the most—in our self-control.

If TV can inspire violence in children, as has been indisputably proven, it can probably also inspire gluttony in adults. Turning a nation of people into instant slobs will not grab the public

174

attention or arouse the type of indignation that turning them into rapists or gunslingers would. And rightly so. But for compulsive eaters it is a matter of major concern. Are food addicts usually TV addicts as well (and vice versa)? Were they fat before they glued themselves to the tube? Is there a relationship between how much television they watch and how much extra weight they carry? How vulnerable are viewers to the images that flit across the omnipresent screens in living rooms, bedrooms, and kitchens? In what ways can it undermine a dieter's resolve, or prevent a Stay Thin candidate from sticking to his guns and turning to candy instead?

It was more than two thousand years ago that the Trojan warrior Paris learned that by striking Achilles in the heel, he could destroy him. Today, the expression "Achilles' heel" means a person's fatal weakness. The chink in his armor. His soft spot.

For many people, television is their Achilles' heel. They can make it through mealtimes, coffee breaks, even parties without succumbing to snackitis. But when they sit down in front of the glass box, they're goners.

Now I have nothing against TV—I have a few favorite programs myself—but a steady diet of sitting and watching can undermine even a strong-willed dieter. First, the physical act of watching keeps him on his duff, when that duff might do very well with a good workout. (Gary H. rides his exercise machine while he watches his favorite shows. That might work for you, if you live alone.

But if there's anyone else trying to watch at the same time, you might get a lot of flack.)

Secondly, prolonged sitting makes a person restless. It's only natural to get up and take a walk—and given the food images on the screen, it's not surprising when that walk leads to the kitchen. And the messages are so enticing. Just as your hair can never be as shiny, or your skin as glowy, so your cooking can never be as mouth-watering or perfect-looking as what you see on TV. But you're tempted to try. And unfortunately, food commercials usually only depict high-calorie foods—cakes, pies, pizza, spaghetti. How many commercials have you seen urging you to eat carrots, lean meat, or fresh fruit?

One patient found it helpful to tune in occasionally to wretched programs like *The $1.98 Beauty Show* or *The Gong Show* to remind herself of the type of respect we accord fat people in our society. "I also keep telling myself that I'm not as bad as they are; but I will be if I keep eating," she chuckled.

But television is not the only trap lying in wait for the unwary dieter, although it's probably the most lethal and pervasive one. Certain times of the day can also be a spur to snacking.

Sally B., a freelance artist who works at home, says her Achilles' Heel is "the elevenses." Though she's careful to eat a nourishing beakfast, she gets hungry, out-of-sorts, and restless about eleven every morning, just as—theoretically—she's deep in her work.

"My Aunt Catherine used to have a glass of

176

port every morning at eleven," Sally remembers. "When I was a little girl, I'd often visit her at that time of day. She'd always give me a glass of ginger ale and a cookie. I vowed that when I grew up, I'd have port like she did too. But I have a very low tolerance for alcohol, besides which my husband would be very alarmed if I told him I had a drink in the morning. So I snack. I think the food does the same thing for me that the wine did for her: makes me high."

Changing meal hours often works to reduce snacking, because when your stomach says it is hungry may be the time for you to eat instead of snack. What Sally finally did, instead of snacking at eleven, was to eat an early lunch, around eleven-thirty. Since the snacking desire was only a serious problem in the late morning, she could then easily get through until dinner time without stopping to eat what she shouldn't.

While changing meal hours works well for some snacking urges, it doesn't work that well with TV. Most of us have gotten used to watching television at the same time: after-breakfast talk shows; after-lunch soap operas; and after-dinner sit-coms and specials. If possible, it's not a bad idea to see if you can combine a meal with those visual orgies. But if that won't work for you, you might try the following.

SET A TIME LIMIT ON SNACKING
Instead of getting up for a snack whenever you feel like it, decide in advance exactly when you're going to take your food break, the later the better

so that a little bit of food doesn't tease you into wanting more. So if you generally watch TV from eight until eleven, decide in advance that you're going to snack only at ten.

GRADUALLY CUT DOWN THE QUANTITY OF SNACKS CONSUMED AS WELL AS THE FREQUENCY OF SNACKING

If you always eat a candy bar during the news, cut down to three-quarters of a candy bar for the next few nights, then down to half a bar, and finally down to a quarter of a bar every third or fourth night.

What do you do with the rest of the candy? Rhoda reduced her intake from a Milky Way a day to a bar of chocolate a week by switching to Hershey Bars, breaking them into squares, wrapping and freezing each one, and then eating only a square every few days when the urge to snack was too strong to resist.

SHAPE THE SNACKS YOU EAT

It is possible also to shape the kind of snacks you eat. Chances are that you now snack mainly on junk foods. So add one low-calorie low-sugar food, such as raw vegetables, to your break. Little by little, increase the number of these nonfattening healthy foods while decreasing the quantity of sweets, until the only snacks you take in are those which are good for you.

Although right now you may be going *argh,* as your experiment progresses, you'll probably learn to like the taste of the natural food better than you did the sweet. Honest. Remember what A. S. Neill said: we are not born with a taste for the wrong things—it is cultivated. (As explained in chapter six, partially by serving as a reward when you were young, food came to satisfy more than just your taste buds.) What we are born with is an instinctive ability to select a good, balanced diet for ourselves. We have simply been programmed to like junk. Deprogram yourself.

DON'T SNACK IN THE KITCHEN

I can't emphasize enough how important it is *not* to eat in the kitchen, in the midst of the cornucopia of plenty. "There I was in the kitchen," recalled Michele G., "starving in the middle of a banquet, with my cup of broth and my crackers. So of course I got up and went to the refrigerator to see what I could find."

Set aside one place, such as the dining room, for at-home snacks as well as meals. Too often we tend to think of snack calories as being less significant than the "real" calories contained in meals. We also minimize just how much snacking we really do, because when we do it all over the house, we don't really get an idea of how much we're stuffing ourselves.

PUT SNACKS DIRECTLY ON A PLATE

Put the food you're going to snack on directly on a plate. NO taking the box of crackers to the table with you because it is very hard to limit quantities when potato chips, pretzels, and crackers are eaten directly from the package. Somehow it always seems as if you're eating less when the food isn't set out in front of you and that makes it harder to realize just how much gorging you're really doing.

SNACK ON THE RIGHT THINGS

And finally, you can allow yourself umlimited TV snacking—but only of the right foods. For example, one of the reasons almost everyone disdains snacks of celery and carrots is because of the burden of cleaning and cutting them up. Make that problem a bonus for you by using the commercials to chop, clean, and ultimately eat these items, rather than dipping into a bag of potato chips at each break.

Most of these suggestions will help control all snacking, and not just the TV munchies: be aware of when you're snacking, try to combine snacks with meals, set time limits, cut down on the quantity, gradually shape the snacks into healthy ones, snack in one place, on a plate, and try to snack on the right things.

So much as is practicable, try to follow these methods in your office as well. If you're going to snack at work, choose your snacks wisely, and don't leave home without them. A lot of overweight people like to enjoy "the pause that refreshes" from the office vending machines. Plus candy. Cookies. And whatever. But that candy bar goes down so fast you hardly know you ate it. And afterwards, that hint of a sweet taste teases you until you buy another one.

On the other hand, if you prepare the right snacks at home and bring them into the office, they are ultimately more satisfying because you have to chew such things as raw cauliflower or string beans. They're also better for your teeth, and won't give you the guilts, those nagging, hateful feelings that make it harder to stick to your regimen because you feel that you've already lost half the battle.

Divide the snacks up the night before, so you won't eat everything at once and then find yourself vaulting over the desk to get to the cookie-vending machine when the second fit hits. Many offices have refrigerators in which employees can stash their "brown bags" of lunch or snacks. But if yours doesn't, don't use that as an excuse. Just bring snacks that need no refrigeration like a small apple, some Ry-Krisps, raisins, etc. And remember to avoid the coffee wagon when it comes around (that's a good time to go to the bathroom), or all of the above could be in vain.

In addition to office snacking, "social" snacking can be a trial by fire for dieters. Mary H. told one of our behavior modification groups that "it got to be so hard to say no when my hostess shoved a tray of hors d'oeuvres at me, that while I was trying to Stay Thin, I stopped going out altogether." But you really don't have to go to such extremes. Simply learn that you can be sociable without having to eat.

Of course for some people this can be very difficult, especially if social eating becomes part of their job. For example, Jack O. was an insurance agent who often visited his clients at home, sometimes making as many as five visits a day. When clients knew he was coming, they would usually prepare coffee and cake for him. Not wanting to hurt their feelings, and concerned about not antagonizing any of them, he rarely said no.

After yo-yoing for years, he finally realized that he would have to discipline himself. So he frankly told the people that while their cake looked delicious, he was watching his weight. Then he would ask for a cup of black coffee or some bouillon.

You'll find, as Jack did, that people are *not* insulted when you reject their offers of food, if you explain that you're genuinely concerned about your weight. Most people are fighting this problem themselves to some degree, and will admire your self-control. But be firm in your refusal. None of this "well, maybe just a sliver" stuff.

The most important thing in controlling any kind of snacking is to be aware that there's a problem and, if possible, to know when it's likely to manifest itself. Is there some part of your day, some chore perhaps that you dread or dislike, that may be regularly catapulting you into a snack? Is there a particular holiday, or perhaps a social function (the office parties maybe), that causes you to have the kind of anxiety that would make a drinker get blotto? Or do you just get the usual 4 P.M. "blahs" like so many people, or the 5-6 P.M. "up-the-wall" syndrome that marks what so many young mothers find is the disintegration hour (when you'll wolf down the leavings on the kids' plates just to spare yourself the trouble of scraping them into the garbage can)?

Find the problem. Then look for the answer. Set your sights high, but don't expect immediate solutions. If you've ever studied anything—a language, mathematics, sculpture—you know that there are periods when you seem to be making enormous strides, followed by other times when you seem to be making no progress at all, or worse still, even seem to be going backwards.

Some people get so discouraged when they hit these "plateaus" that they quit—but that's a shame. Accept the fact that plateaus are inevitable, and that when you get through them, you'll be able to go on to another period of progress.

You won't always have to be a slave to snacks.

11
Changing the Way You Eat

Until now, we've focused mainly on ways to understand and change the pattern of your life so that Staying Thin can supplant your previous pastime of Constantly Going On Another Diet. Now we are ready to move on to specifics of Staying Thin.

These next few chapters will show you some physical ways to change your world, a process absolutely as important as the psychological refocusing you've started to learn from the earlier chapters. (Some of those changes won't happen overnight, but you'll be amazed at how much input will reemerge as you work on Staying Thin.)

It would be nice if these changes weren't necessary. But you are confronted with food temptations so continually, that unless you change some of your habits, there is no way that you will be able to keep your weight down.

Eating is an oral addiction that's much harder to conquer than smoking or drinking. Indeed, ex-smokers and former drinkers may have an easier time because what they give up, they give up entirely. No exceptions. The rule is inflexible. And to a considerable degree its very rigidity makes it easier to follow than the more tractable rules that govern the constant "what," "when," and "how much" choices that the compulsive overeater must learn to make.

You can quit cigarettes cold turkey and never buy another pack. You can stop drinking and never pick up another glass. Furthermore, if you choose your friends carefully, you may rarely be tempted by watching other people smoke and drink right in front of you. But there's no way you can just quit eating or stop being confronted by food. (If you live alone, you can mold your environment so as to avoid watching others eat forbidden goodies, but even that's hard).

As a result, breaking a smoking or drinking habit requires superior discipline, but breaking the overeating habit requires almost superhuman restraint. The smoker or drinker can avoid his poison; the overeater must confront his downfall several times a day. There is no way to stop eating by going cold turkey. Naturally, you can give up snacking, desserts, or cocktail goodies, because those are optional anyway. But you are still constantly confronted with food, and if a compulsive eater gets started on even a small portion, he or she usually winds up devouring the whole of whatever it was.

Visual cues for food—omnipresent in our environment—are a constant temptation to overweight persons. The very sight of food, or even its photographic image, is enough to make them think they're starving. We all know how ads for food on television, displays in pastry shops, or a baked Alaska being served at the next restaurant table can affect us.

It would be nice if you could go to a desert island for a few months, where you would never be tempted by the sight of forbidden food, or set off by a clock that reminds you that it's lunch hour. Then, on the day that you reach your magic number (your goal weight), a boat would come from the mainland to take you home.

Actually, some people do do a form of this. Remember Sally S., whose husband gave her a present each year of a week at a "fat farm"? In these fantasy-type places—as unlike the real world as Mars—the patients' daily bread is doled out to them in crumbs. They have no access to a kitchen or a town with edible temptations. And three times a day, they go to the dining room and stare glumly at a plate containing a couple of ounces of fish, a narrow wedge of lemon, and invariably a large sprig of parsley.

And they do lose weight, but without unlearning their self-destructive behavior. The spa-owners know that they can count on these ladies' return business. They'll be back. Running away—or behaving for a week—is not the answer to a lifetime eating problem.

Some people choose even greater extremes in

their attempt to escape from the problem of food. Suzy C., who did not have the money to go to a "fat farm," simply stayed home. Always. "I knew that if I went to a party, a restaurant, or even to a friend's house, I'd eat," she explained simply.

Suzy stuck to her diet all right, but she was also miserable. Cut off from her social life, eating a brown-bag lunch at her office desk every day instead of going out with the girls, life became drab indeed. In fact, Suzy was one of the few patients who entered our program thin—but miserable. Her goal—which she accomplished—was to learn the difference between discipline and deprivation.

Perhaps the following suggestions will at first seem a bit like deprivation, but it won't take long—often just a couple of months of regularly following these suggestions—before they become second nature and simple lifelong habits that make the difference between where you are now and Thin City. Even though you've heard some of these ideas before, as you read them, think afresh of how you could incorporate all of them into your daily routine.

To lose weight, and to Stay Thin as well, you have to eat less. It may seem obvious, but that doesn't make it any less true. Later, we'll discuss strategies for making meals taste better, last longer, and satisfy more. But for now, I want to emphasize that the best way to cut down on the actual amount of food you consume is to eat only when you're hungry. We've already gone over some techniques to help you control extra-curricular bingeing and snacking but you must learn to listen to your stomach at mealtimes as well.

Just because it's "dinner time" doesn't mean it's dinner time. If it's seven o'clock and dinner is served, that still doesn't mean you have to eat it. Ask yourself, "Am I really hungry?" And if you're not, just eat a little, and don't feel that you have to have a full meal just because the clock—or your family—says it's time. If you skip the meal now, you can allow yourself something later on—when you are hungry.

Sure this kind of discipline can be tough if you have to sit at the table while others eat. One way to cope is to keep a long cool drink beside you and take small sips throughout the meal. (Actually, this will accomplish more than just helping you through the ordeal. A University of Maryland study recently showed that six-ten glasses of water, unsugared iced tea, or other nonsugary liquid consumed daily, helped stave off hunger pangs because people often confuse feelings of thirst with feelings of hunger).

You should also tailor your lunch hour to your stomach's needs. Somebody once decided that noon was the time for lunch, but it is not written on a stone tablet and handed down from on high. Often, noon is three hours or so after breakfast, (when you're not really ready for another meal), and seven or eight hours away from dinner—too long to wait.

Changing your meal patterns is not as difficult as you think. Horace H., for example, was a sales executive with a large Michigan furniture concern. He was constantly having to entertain clients at lunch—but he was a breakfast person. The high point of his eating day came just a few minutes after he jumped out of bed in the morning. He needed and enjoyed big breakfasts, and found he couldn't stop snacking all morning without suffering a lack of energy during the working day.

So, when lunchtime came around, and for business reasons he had to eat with his clients, there was Horace, sitting across a restaurant table from them, flanked by a dry martini, and a basket of bread, neither of which he particularly wanted. But they were there so he ate them. And he began to gain weight, as well as feel tired, logy, and lacking in energy during the afternoons. He was simply eating more than he wanted or needed.

Horace found a way out of his trap: he began meeting clients for breakfast, or for an early brunch. They ate less, and they certainly drank less. And Horace went back to his usual program—just right for him—of a solid meal in the morning and another in the evening, without the heavy lunch and drinks, unneeded and unwanted, in between.

Most of you, like Pavlov's dogs salivating at the sound of the bell, are ready to eat when the clock tells you the hour has come. You no longer bother to listen to your stomach. And so, your ability to perceive real hunger has gotten all bollixed up. Like a blind man tapping his way down a street, and straining to get a sense of what is in his path, you're dependent on external cues. Habit, psychological craving, and conformity play a larger role in your eating habits than you realize.

Sticking to a standard schedule divorces you from the actual promptings of your stomach. And when you don't know what your stomach really needs, and when it needs it, you're all the more likely to overfeed it.

Need I say more?

Another way to listen to your stomach is to concentrate solely on the food when you're eating. One of the reasons you overate was that most of the time you didn't even realize you were stuffing your mouth, probably because other parts of your body were doing other things (often a habit unconsciously cultivated to keep you from realizing just how much you are piling in). Your mind may have been thousands of miles away. Your eyes may have been riveted on a television set, a magazine, or a book. Or, in between bites, you were talking to someone at the table—or worse still, on the telephone.

For now, you are just going to concentrate totally on what you're eating. First, that will make you enjoy it more so that you can derive more pleasure from less food. Second, it will give you the opportunity to gauge whether you're eating past the point of hunger. (You've got to listen to your stomach when it says "thanks, but no thanks.") You can't do all this at once. When you have to watch your weight, you can't do two (or more) things simultaneously if one of them is eating. That means no watching TV, no reading the latest Barbara Cartland, no gossiping with friends, etc., while you're eating. You're all too likely to just keep pushing the food down as long as it's there.

Some people will go along with banning the TV from the table, but feel that there's nothing wrong with getting in some more studying or reading along with their meat and potato (oops, I mean meat and salad). Sue G., who's addicted to mystery stories (and to eating while she's reading them), complained that when she gets into one of them, she simply can't stop—even for meals. "I've got to know who did it," she wailed. That's understandable, but if she wants to lose weight, she'll just have to wait until some time other than while she's eating to uncover the murderer. Otherwise, she may very well do herself in.

"But I'm not reading for fun, Doctor," Maxine G. protested. "I just have to study all the time during my twice-a-year exams or I'll get an *F*." But if she studies while she's eating, she will definitely get an *F*—for fat.

There are simply no excuses acceptable in this area, and believe me, as a bariatric physician, I've heard them all.

One other thing that will help you concentrate solely on your eating is not to eat on the run. Maria N., an editor at a publishing house, habitually ate her lunch at her desk, wolfing down the food so as to get on with what she thought were more important things. As a result, she would be hungry an hour or two later, and would telephone for another sandwich, or salivate at the sound of the coffee-wagon bell.

Despite the fact that she'd always considered herself a wiry person, Maria suddenly discovered the telltale signs of middle-aged spread—at the age of thirty-two. She's learned to recognize this destructive eating behavior, and now gives time to the eating process.

No matter how busy you are, at work, or around the house, you should set aside enough time to eat. Eating on the run ultimately leads to excessive, unaware eating. Too many Americans gulp down a sandwich at their desks, at the wheels of their cars, or on the street. Look at the proliferation of hotdog wagons and other food carts on any big city street. Those vendors cater to people who don't want to spend time eating. But look also at the weight of many of the people who stop there.

Figure out a way to make your lunch hour, or half hour, or whatever, a time that you set aside totally for eating. Slow, pleasant eating will relax you, and give you energy which will allow you to "make up for lost time" in the afternoon.

Also, try not to eat at your desk if you can find an alternative place. Sitting somewhere else—even in someone else's office—will help break the connection between your desk and food, and make it harder for you to eat and do something else at the same time: read, make phone calls, take notes, etc. All of the practices you follow at home are just as important in the office.

SLOW DOWN YOUR EATING
To have the opportunity to listen to your stomach,

the most important thing you can do is to slow down your eating. I'm sure you've heard before that it takes about twenty minutes for the stomach to signal the brain that it's full—but repetition doesn't make it any less true.

If one simple change in habit was to do the most to help you stay slim, it would be this one. In fact, if you don't believe that fast eaters are fat eaters, just look around the next time you're at a dinner party. The fattest people always finish before the thinner ones (and then beg for seconds). The skinnies, on the other hand, will seem to dawdle, will appear to even forget the food is there, will push it around with their forks, and will leave some of it over on their plate, especially if their portion was large. But chances are, even though you'll eat at least two times more than they will, you'll finish sooner and leave an empty plate. And it isn't—as you've no doubt convinced yourself—because you're physically hungrier, or your larger stomach needs more food.

That slowing down your eating slows down your progress towards obesity is proven in studies as well. A recent research survey of children in a school cafeteria showed that thin children did take smaller bites, and stopped eating more often to put down their utensils. The fatties just dug in, shoveling in their food, and pausing for nothing until they were satiated. Still another study of adults yielded much the same results, and proved additionally that fatter people take larger bites and chew only half as many times as thinner people.

Maybe you've been wolfing down your food so

that you won't feel so guilty about eating, maybe feeling that if you get it over with quickly, you aren't really eating that much. Or, while it's unlikely that you would confess it to yourself, your need for immediate gratification may be so intense that you just can't wait. Even worse, maybe you're just plain greedy and want to make sure that you get yours before the food runs out. While you're unlikely to admit to yourself that you're so covetous, it may help to slow you down if you realize that others with better manners will think that, or the worst about you, when they see you piling in the food at what is to them an alarming rate.

An easy, rather amusing way to note the difference between gluttony and polite eating is to watch a dog and a cat at feeding time. Generally, the dog will eat every morsel as fast as he can from the moment the dish touches the floor in front of him. But the fastidious feline, though he may have been meowing for his food for half an hour, will usually approach his dish slowly and serenely, take a few bites, and then go off and do whatever cats do. Sometimes, he'll return casually to finish the meal later; notice too that if you try to interrupt a dog while he's eating, if you don't get a bite you'll at least get a menacing growl. But the cat is more casual; if you interrupt his dinner, it's no big deal.

When you think about it, the habit of eating rapidly and without pauses does look terrible to others—unless you're a dog. Do you want people to think you're nervous, greedy, unable to control yourself, etc? Think about that the next time you start to wolf down a meal in front of others, if you're unable to slow down for the sake of Staying Thin.

The following are a few tricks to slow down your eating, if voluntary self-restraint isn't your thing.

Before you begin to eat, cut your food into really small pieces. Not only will it take more time to eat all the tiny morsels, but the act of cutting the food will itself occupy some of the moments that you might have used for eating it.

Play the old dieter's trick of slowing the pace of a meal by laying down your fork or spoon between bites.

To stretch a meal out, pat your mouth with your napkin at frequent intervals. Besides slowing you down, and giving you time to check on whether you're really full, it also makes you look terribly polite.

Really chew each bite before swallowing it. Most likely you'll find that you've been swallowing great unchewed lumps of food. Try to be dainty; eat morsels, not gobs.

One of my patients, Janet S., found it helpful to prop a small mirror in front of her when she was eating alone. It showed her how fast she was really eating (we usually don't have the opportunity to see this), gave her an indication of how bad she looked to others, and when she decided to change, watching herself slowly chewing the food made it easier for it to become second nature to her.

Finish the food that's already in your mouth before stuffing any more in. It sounds basic, but take note the next time you eat. You probably don't do it.

Taking only one kind of food in each mouthful will probably make you eat more slowly. Compulsive eaters get into bad habits like spearing a piece of meat, dipping it into the mashed potatoes, and then topping it with a few green peas if they can. A wine taster does't confuse his palate with an assortment of wines in one gulp. Neither does someone who really wants to be able to taste the food. Which brings us to the next point.

Work at really tasting and enjoying each bite. You might try Cheryl H.'s method which is to chew all food for any meal only on one side of her mouth. She says that heightens her sensitivity to the food's taste and if you get more taste out of your food, it's a fact that you'll need to eat less of it. When you learn to taste your food, you go slower, the better to savor it. You are also then better able to sense the moment you are full. You're not only able to listen to your stomach but to hear its answer.

James Beard aside, how many fat gourmet cooks have you seen? The reason is that skinny people and gourmets (how often the two go together) know how to *really* taste the food, savor the bouquet, and study the aftertaste. One cook who is now permanently thin (it appears) revealed that the difference between the way she ate when she was a gourmand and the way she eats these days as a gourmet, is that "now I concentrate on chewing and tasting my food. When I was fat, I used to concentrate on swallowing it." Or, put another way, one fifty-pound loser—or should I say winner—admitted that "I never observed the quality or quantity of what I was eating. I just ate."

Before eating dessert wait fifteen minutes to give your stomach time to signal the brain that you're full. If you are, you might want to "save" it, and have it several hours later, thereby cutting out one of your more likely snacks.

The final two pointers to be made here now are not ways to stretch out a meal but to shrink it, in other words, to eat less. First, decide now that instead of always eating every single morsel on your plate, you're always going to leave some food over. In fact, some of the worst offenders are not only those who clean their own plates but others' plates as well.

Lucienda, a clean-plate fiend from the time she was a child, would cook and serve supper at five-thirty to her three young children, before she ate her own dinner. If they failed to clean their plates (as children frequently do) Lucienda would do it for them. "I just can't bring myself to scrape perfectly good food into the garbage," she rationalized.

She now scrapes the kids' leftovers into the dog's dish and everyone—including the dog—is happier.

Arlene D. started to put on weight when her children were toddlers. She was fine until they were two years old, since the food they ate earlier didn't appeal to her very much anyway. After all, who has a craving for mashed bananas? But then, in the normal course of childhood, they went through a period of not being interested in food. "I thought I wasn't a good mother unless I made those full meals anyway, just in case," she said. "And then I was left with half-eaten peanut butter and jelly sandwiches, scrambled eggs, ravioli and more. I became a garbage can for what they didn't eat."

It took years for Arlene to finally solve her problem (the children grew older, which helped). Now, they clear the table and dispose of whatever they leave on their plates. And they also take out the garbage when they're finished, leaving no odd cookie crumbs to tempt their as yet weak-willed mother.

As to leaving food over on your own plate, yes, it's still true: there are people starving in Europe, not to mention America. But eating everything on your plate is not going to help them one iota—and look at how damaging that kind of behavior has been to you. Many members of yesterday's Clean-Plate Club are today trying to Stay Thin. As

Hiram C. said ruefully, "I've got this starving-in-India syndrome. I'm fifty-nine years old, and I haven't noticed that less people are starving after a lifetime of overeating."

If you are really concerned about the starving people in other parts of the world, don't have an Eat-in but do make a donation to an appropriate charity. And treat yourself kindly by unlearning your clean-plate compulsion. Cultivate the leaving of food on your plate. "Leave some for Miss Manners," some grandmothers used to say.

But more than just politeness is at stake. Remember that eating every last bite is compulsive behavior, and that kind of behavior is what made you overweight in the first place. As you've gone through life, you've taken whatever people dished out to you. Literally. At restaurants, you ate the entire platter. ("It costs money; I can't throw it out.") At dinner parties, you ate whatever the hostess gave you. ("I don't like it, but I don't want to insult her.") Even when you served yourself, you doled out gargantuan portions. ("That'll keep me from having seconds," but most of the time you went back for more anyway.)

Your signal to stop eating was that your plate was empty. But if you want to Stay Thin, you have to learn that the signal to stop eating is when your stomach is full. For the first time since you started having weight problems, you have to start paying attention to whether or not you're hungry *before* taking the next bite. Remember what we discussed earlier: most of what you thought was hunger was a psychological craving for food, and not a physiological one.

Another point, and one I've already touched upon in this chapter, is that the only way you're going to be able to control yourself at meals, and not overdo things, is to teach yourself that when you do feel full you stop eating. A catch phrase of contemporary "pop psychology" is to "get in touch with your feelings." Well, every overweight person who wants to be thin has to get in touch with his stomach's feelings. He has to learn to sense when his stomach (not his mind or emotions) needs food. And he has to learn to sense when his stomach has had enough.

Of course, if, as we discussed earlier, he's actively working to make his life richer, through sports, hobbies, and intellectual pursuits, his mind and emotions will be somewhat distracted from food. But the bad habits of many years are not that easily broken, I'm afraid. And new habits, new sensitivities must be cultivated.

Ironically, there are people who suffer from a disturbance called anorexia nervosa, which is the reverse of your problem. Anorexics are so hyperaware of the feeling of fullness that, taking in even a very small amount of food seems to produce in them an immediate and usually uncomfortable feeling of being stuffed.

Compulsive eaters go in the opposite direction (although thankfully, not as severely), and have trouble knowing when they are full, usually letting an empty plate, rather than their stomach, signal the end of eating.

So it's time to sharpen your awareness of feeling

full. Don't be like Norton S., who, ever since he got divorced, eats in restaurants—a real trap to begin with anyway. He makes it worse by eating in Italian restaurants, although usually the same one. He peruses the menu, then decides that "tonight I'll restrain myself. I'll just have the ravioli and a green salad."

That's a bad choice to begin with, but the situation is made worse when the waiter arrives at the table (who knows Norton by now) and suggests that the veal is unusually tender tonight, "just the way you like it," he assures his prey. Norton invariably decides that he'll "splurge tonight and diet tomorrow" and then orders that, along with the ravioli and salad.

And then, after the ravioli, and while waiting for his veal, he has some bread and butter along with some vegetables. Later there's dessert too—which Norton wouldn't think of skipping since it comes with the meal. He probably really feels full long before he ends his meal, but he never stops to listen to his stomach, or to ask himself what more he really needs. Instead, after overordering in the first place, he always thinks to himself, "As long as I've paid for it, it's a sin not to eat it."

But the real sin is what has happened to his body. And the pity of it is that the situation could so easily have been controlled if Norton had just paused periodically to honestly gauge whether or not he was still hungry, and then stopped as soon as he knew he wasn't.

So, to get back in touch with your stomach, and

actually eat less, start listening—to yourself, to your needs. Don't eat by the clock, don't eat while you're doing something else, slow down your eating with the suggestions above, make your meals last longer, start to really taste your food, and when you feel full, STOP.

The following points will also help you Stay Thin by changing the way you serve and prepare meals.

SET THE SCENE
Some psychologists suggest that you try to make every meal as pleasant as possible in order to derive more pleasure from the food while eating less. By using good dinnerware, tablecloths, or pretty placemats, linen napkins, fresh flowers, and so on, you make eating a festive occasion.

Work on making the food look more attractive as well. You'll feel better after eating meals that have a built-in visual appeal.

We all remember (how can we forget?) some institution, school, camp, or whatever we attended, where certain of the meals were absolutely hateful looking. Usually we found unflattering nicknames for these dishes, most of which can't be repeated here. Mary S. giggles as she recalls Sunday dinner at YMCA camp. "It was all white," she remembers, "Chicken, mashed potatoes, a creamy gravy, cauliflower, milk, and vanilla ice cream. Yuck."

Be aware of color, texture, and variety, and learn to enjoy your meals visually as well as gastronomically. The women's magazines are full of tips for meals that have eye appeal—but leave out the high calorie decorations.

DON'T TASTE WHILE PREPARING FOOD

For many people, the hardest time is not in between meals, but right before the meal—during preparation—when the anticipation level is highest. This is the time when you have to see, smell, and touch food without actually eating it. It's a time when temptation is lying in your path, when you're usually alone, and when you have none of the distractions that you have during the actual meal. Simply rule out tasting and allow no exceptions. Someone else in the family will probably be more than happy to taste it to see if it's right for you.

I don't suggest going this far, but Maxine B., who was married to a doctor, got one of his surgical masks and kept it over her nose and mouth while she was cooking to help keep the enticing smells out of her nostrils and her food-gathering fingers out of her mouth.

NEVER EAT IN THE KITCHEN

Since the very sight (not to mention smell and touch) of food can metamorphose you into the Mad Eater, resolve to eat in the dining room, at least until you have reeducated your responses. If you have no dining room, set up a small dining area in your living room—but away from the TV. Eat everything—even snacks—in that area.

It's good to always confine all your eating to one place anyway, since this limits the number of cues for eating. For example, Donna used to like to bring a lot of little snacks out to the backyard when she was doing her gardening. The problem was that after a while, doing gardening became a cue to snack.

This also often happens when you eat all around the house. Watch TV/have some food. Sit in one chair/drink a martini. Lie on the couch/have a candy bar. After a while, there are so many cues that are hard to control, your eating goes out of control as well.

Besides which, if you eat all over the house, you often don't realize just how much you're eating, since we tend only to count as "food" what we eat in the dining room. Eating in only one place may help you realize just how much you're eating without being aware of it.

Also, when possible, don't eat alone in this area. People who eat alone are often tempted to do other things to keep them occupied, such as reading or watching television. Secondly, to put it bluntly, you're more likely to cheat when you're by yourself. So, even if you live alone, try to eat with someone else (preferably someone who will support you weight-wise) as often as possible.

DON'T SERVE BUFFET STYLE MEALS
Interesting arrays of food, arranged on platters, invite you to grab, and are therefore too tempting for most people with chronic weight problems. The impulse to refill is also too strong when the extra food is right in front of you. So, fill your plate in the kitchen, and carry it into the dining area.

And don't look back.

MAKE THE PORTIONS LOOK BIGGER

The easiest way to do this is to buy smaller dinner plates (most are nine inches, so buy the seven-inch size). If you don't want to buy a new set of dishes, use paper plates (which come in seven-inch sizes), or use your salad plates for the main course. But don't try to force this plan on other members of your family, or on guests. One man whose wife had held her weight at 116 for over six months grouched that "she looks great, but my food keeps falling off the edges of those little plates."

Here are a few other ways to make portions look larger by making the plate seem fuller.

Buy parsley or watercress and pile it around the edges of your plate.

Put your food on beds of lettuce, and, of course, eat the lettuce after you're finished.

Spread the food around. Say you're having three thin slices of roast beef for lunch. Instead of having the three on top of each other (which is the way they come wrapped from the deli), spread the slices around. Not only will it look like more food, but it will take you longer to eat it. Which is another one of your goals.

CHANGE THE ORDER OF WHAT YOU EAT

Be flexible. What order you eat food in generally makes very little difference to most people, but anything that makes compulsives more aware of the food while they're eating is helpful. One of the men in our classes, Jim W., reports success in ranking the food on his plate according to calories. He eats the lowest calorie food first, then the next highest, and so on. By leaving the highest calorie food for last, his stomach is often full when he reaches it, and he is sometimes able to pass it up entirely.

A variation of this is to eat the salad first, which most people nibble at with their entrees. Eating it first helps stretch out the time you spend eating.

Establish your own order—and vary it at times. One trick, which I'm not sure I would recommend, but which Paul S. swears by, is eating dessert first. He says dieting makes him feel deprived, and dessert is what he feels most deprived of. So he makes himself feel good first; then the low calorie dishes in the rest of the meal have less importance to him. He also finds that he can eat more slowly this way, because he's less anxious to race through his meal so he can dive into his favorite dessert.

BEWARE THE BEFORE DINNER DRINK

Even if your diet allows you to drink, remember that alcohol often weakens your resolve—and spurs your appetite. Harold found it helpful when he was in a restaurant to stop having a cocktail before deciding what to have for dinner, because when he did he usually ordered more than he had planned to when he first entered the restaurant. Now he sits down and asks for a menu, orders his entire meal, and *then* orders his drink.

If you must drink, and your diet allows it, try a white-wine spritzer instead of a regular hard

206

drink. This half-and-half combination of dry white wine and club soda contains only about seventy-five calories, considerably fewer than most other drinks, and stretched by the club soda to a good size you will be able to sip it slowly and make it last for some time.

DIET COOKING AND NUTRITION

Staying thin does not mean giving up eating. But learning to distinguish among foods must become your first line of defense. So replace the villains of your old diet with a whole new cast of good guys.

Ever notice that fattening foods have a certain something that makes them physically satisfying? They're gooey . . . crunchy . . . crackly . . . thick. You can eat them with your hands, and they're designed to be easily transportable to your mouth. They come in bags and boxes and don't have to be prepared, giving you extra time to eat it all.

Who needs it?

Attempt to make friends with so-called diet foods. Try things you think you "hate," and make sure it's not just the idea that troubles you rather than the actual taste. Keep an open mind, and try to forget that these foods are dietetic.

Sometimes, you can reeducate your taste by patient work. Maybe you're one of those people, for instance, who can't stand the taste of low-fat cottage cheese. So mix some of the higher-fat kind with the low-fat type and continue to vary the proportions until you have gotten used to the lower-fat cottage cheese.

Or make cottage cheese creamier by mixing it

with a little plain, low-fat yogurt. Or give skim milk more body by mixing nonfat dry milk solids into it. Some people would rather have a small glass of refreshing delicious whole milk than two big glasses of skim milk which one patient calls "gray milk." "Ugh," she says. "No matter how hard and long I try, I can't get used to drinking that stuff, much less looking at it." All right, you don't have to like everything.

Others can't tolerate the idea of margarine (some still call it "oleo," remembering the days when it looked like lard until you stirred the capsule of yellow coloring into it. *Then* it was bad). But you can learn to accept diet margarine and diet mayonnaise by experimenting with different brands and mixing different amounts into food until you build up a tolerance.

In general, develop some awareness of calories and nutrition. Understand the type of damage that your old food was doing to your body. Know the caloric cost of things. For example, you can eat a giant bowl of salad for less than one hundred calories—but if you add just one tablespoon of dressing, you may be more than doubling the caloric cost of the salad. Learn to use your calories better so you can eat more of what you want without feeling that you're depriving yourself. If you're unhappy, and wallow in self-pity, you won't Stay Thin for long.

You should learn something about the calorie content of low-calorie foods as well. Cottage cheese, for example, varies widely from maker to maker. Some brands have 4 percent milkfat; while others have only ½ of 1 percent. (Many food manufacturers print the calorie content of foods right on the package.)

Instead of feeling sorry for yourself that your new regimen is "boring," and worse still, fantasizing about now permanently forbidden foods, learn to add zest to your new diet with spices and seasonings. They're low in calories (or contain none at all) and can make your food taste far more interesting so you'll be happier with smaller portions (and taste it better). There are lots of condiment cookbooks around that will give you ideas about how to spice up almost any dish.

CUT DOWN ON SALT

A simple change in your eating habits, and one that you should make to maintain your health as well as your weight, is to cut down drastically—if not altogether—on the use of ordinary table salt. Besides the fact that it isn't good for you (to over-simplify things a bit), salt makes you retain water so that you'll be more likely to put on weight. Although the weight is not fat, it does have a tendency to discourage you. Anything that makes you feel that things are not going along according to plan could lead you to chuck it all and go back to your old wanton ways.

Most of the time we reach for the salt shaker on the table out of habit anyway, and not out of real desire. As far as bodily need is concerned, people only require *one gram* of salt a day—about one-eighth of a teaspoon. Yet most of us easily eat ten or twenty times that amount.

There are salt substitutes you can try, and a few patients have reported some success with seasoned salt substitutes. Still others have found it helpful to increase their use of pepper, which adds some sharpness and taste to the food, as will a squeeze of lemon, garlic, or other herbs.

To cut down on salt, never salt food before you taste it, try unsalted butter instead of the salted kind, never salt food while it's cooking (not only may some of the salt you put in be unnecessary, but it takes some of the vitamins out of some foods), and remove the shaker from the table altogether (you might wish to replace it with a container of basil leaves or sesame seeds).

You are now at the stage where you can analyze your own patterns and find those small chinks in your dieting armor that have been preventing you from achieving your goal of Staying Thin.

The time to start is at your next meal.

12
Changing Your Environment

Food most often hits you where you live, the very place where you are most likely to let down your defenses, drop your guard, and let habit take over. You probably turn out the lights in the same order every night, switch on the TV news at the same time each day, and set the alarm for the same hour. But those habits that pertain to your eating may be the most ingrained—and may need the most modification. And the best place to start is right in your own backyard.

Or in your kitchen. The purpose of this chapter is to get you to look around at your environment—the place where you live—and see what you could do to make it an easier place in which to Stay Thin.

Most of the changes are simple, and all will work—*if* you actually do them. Just reading about them and nodding your head won't do a thing.

For example, did you *actually* follow that suggestion made in chapter 7 about placing things you
like to do in a strategic spot on the way to the
kitchen? If not, back track and do it now. You
have to follow each of these suggestions if you're
really going to turn your life around at last.

POST PICTURES TO MOTIVATE YOURSELF
First of all, you must always remember where you
came from. And where you want to go. If you
have a snapshot of yourself (which no doubt is
hidden away) from your worst days, dig it out and
have some copies made. Tape one to the
refrigerator, another to the pantry cupboard, a
third on the mirror you use most often. Every few
weeks, alternate them so they jar you into seeing
them again. Don't be embarrassed about other
people seeing them too; most people have padded
skeletons in their closets as well.

A German psychologist has found it best for her
dieting patients for them to actually keep the
photographs alongside their plates at mealtime to
help them slim—one full-length and unflattering
shot and the other showing how they looked in
their youngest, slimmest days.

Don L., on the other hand, had a formerly fat
picture of himself blown up to life size. Then, he
hung it in front of the refrigerator like a curtain so
every time he opens the refrigerator door, he has
to pass it. "That damned thing is as good as an
iron curtain," he says. You don't really have to go
that far; a small snapshot will do the trick for
most people.

Even when it's not in front of you, keep the before and after pictures in your mind and think about it at those moments when someone asks you to play tennis and you're worried about your fat thighs, or during those embarrassing hours at the swimming pool when everyone else seems to look sexy in their suits and trunks.

After you've reached your goal weight, and kept it stable for a while, you may want to throw them out. DON'T. One reason we study history is to teach us of our mistakes so that we won't make them again. Those before pictures are your history; we are all potential recidivists, and must guard against those moments when our reserves fail and we backslide. In addition, it's good to have a reminder of the hard work it took to get you where you are today.

If you really don't want the pictures around when you're slim, you can put them inside cupboards and inside the refrigerator door. You can even make a scrapbook of your before-slim self. But never throw them away or the image may come back to haunt you. Don't try to repress the fact that this is where you were, because, but for the grace of Staying Thin, you would still be there. And if you forget that, you could be back.

"I'd never let anybody take my picture when I was fat," says Harry L. firmly. "As a result, I don't have anything to remind me of those days."

That's no excuse. If this is true for you too, have a full-length photograph taken of you now (unless you're at your fattest), and draw in the old shape on your figure and face with a magic marker as a reminder of what a blob you once let yourself become.

Posting magazine pictures of models and movie stars may also help motivate you. Alana D., on the other hand, felt that she needed an even more graphic reminder. She went out and bought lard, put it in one-pound bags, and placed the bags in her refrigerator. Then, every time she lost a pound, she would put away a bag of lard; every time she gained one, she would add lard to her stock.

She became anxious to get rid of all the lard in the refrigerator (how do you explain *that* to someone?), and seeing the fat she was losing in such literal, visual terms made weight maintenance easier. Such symbolic gestures may seem silly, but if it works, nothing is foolish.

The point here is continued and acute *awareness,* awareness of where you have been, where you are now, and where you plan to go. But note that you must contantly take advantage of these reminders. If you look past your pictures and through your mirrors, they won't do you a damned bit of good.

CHANGES IN THE KITCHEN ITSELF

Anything that encourages you to spend extra time in the kitchen has got to go. So the first thing to do is to take out that phone. And no cheating with phones that have extra long cords which reach into the kitchen. Janet, who lost weight "successfully" eight times, attributed part of Downfall Number Seven to a long extension cord "in case the phone rang while I was cooking." She spent hours in the kitchen calling people she didn't even want to talk to, in some cases didn't even like, because it gave her an excuse to nibble.

Secondly, stop making the kitchen a family center. Most of us have pleasant memories associated with the kitchen, memories that usually date back to our childhood. Even now, being there more often than not gives us a warm good feeling, even independent of food.

Unfortunately, until you're on steadier ground, the kitchen should be a place only for cooking. Not for eating. Or socializing. Get rid of the television set and even the radio. Don't keep family messages in the kitchen; it only encourages everyone to congregate there.

"My children like to do their homework in the kitchen," says Elizabeth J. "They say that the light is better, and they like having a large surface—the kitchen table—to spread their work out on. But when Jackie called me in for a math problem, I always picked up a little something to nibble on while I helped her." Only after she put on thirty-two pounds did she buy each of her children good reading lamps and desks with large tops. They work in their own rooms, now, and if they need her, Elizabeth goes there.

CHANGE THE WAY YOU REFRIGERATE

One place where temptation obviously lurks is in the refrigerator. But just a few simple changes in the way you store foods in there can help you keep from giving in.

Remove, or unscrew the light bulb in the refrigerator to help fight the joy of midnight raids. "Every night, after dinner, I unscrewed the light bulb," a patient admitted in one of our classes. "I still went on midnight raids anyway for a while. Hell, I always knew where everything in the refrigerator was, by heart. But it doesn't seem like the Twinkies are winking up at you when the refrigerator isn't all lit up. Somehow, nothing looks quite as attractive in the dark. I finally got bored with the whole thing and gave up."

The same principle works for wrapping food. If you keep your refrigerator filled with glass see-through jars, and keep items covered with plastic wrap and wax paper, opening up your refrigerator will always be the beginning of the end. Food you can't see is less tempting, and by the time you've unwrapped it, you may have decided against eating it.

The plastic containers that cottage cheese comes in are economical as well as opaque. Bobbie S., who's been using them for two years now (she wraps them with masking tape and then writes on the tape so she knows what's in there), says "When I open the door, all I see are rows of cottage cheese containers—and I don't even like cottage cheese. The very sight is an appetite deterrent."

That what you can't see can't hurt you was proven in an experiment at the University of Pennsylvania cafeteria when gooey fattening desserts were placed at the front of the dessert counter, and the things that are better for everyone in the back. Sure enough, fattening stuff was the first to be taken. But it wasn't just for the reasons you think, because when the two types of desserts were switched around, people tended to reach for the low-calorie high-nutrition food faster.

The next point is to get rid of leftovers before they get rid of you. Unfortunately, we all feel more guilty about throwing out leftovers than we do about overeating, getting fat, and hurting our own bodies (not to mention appearance, morale, etc.) Furthermore, we always seem to manufacture some excuse for keeping these tempting foods around the house—for the dog, for a stew we might make, whatever.

Sometimes, our excuse is somebody else. Sylvia lived with her mother, who was very ill. She had no appetite and had to be coaxed to eat. It was imperative that Sylvia try to get as much food into her mother's mouth as she could. So, one night, she would urge her mother to sip the creamy eggnog which had been sitting on the table for half an hour; the next night it would be the milk shake, and so on.

But despite her daughter's coaxing, Mrs. Smith had little appetite, and never finished anything. Sylvia, on the other hand, didn't feel right about throwing away perfectly good untouched food. So she would finish off the rest.

One day, she and her boyfriend were at an amusement park and they weighed themselves. Sylvia's eyes bulged at the weight increase that had taken place in just a couple of months. That's when she decided that she would have to lose the weight and change her habits so that she could keep it off.

Hers was a real-home-environment-change problem: two people living together, one desperately needing to gain weight, the other passionately wanting to lose it. She solved her problem in three ways. Realizing that her mother was barely touching the food anyway, she started preparing smaller portions. Secondly, she would leave the snack with her mother and not stay to watch it being consumed—or rejected. And when she returned later, and her mother had left most of it, she would quickly throw it away.

These solutions may work for you if you've got a situation where you must prepare food for others. But whenever possible, let others prepare their own snacks. If you're the one who cooks for your family, and you've been doing it for years, it's hard to announce now at this late date that they will become their own cooks (unless you want to start a riot). But you *can* let them know that from now on, they will prepare their own snacks—all between-meal eating. No more making ice cream sodas for your son when he comes home from school. Or laying out all those tempting cheeses to accompany your spouse's drink in the evening.

Don't leave yourself open to finishing up the leftovers in the name of conservation. Here again, a dog would come in handy. But then too, you might end up with a fat dog. Sometimes, my friends, things simply have to be thrown out. Grit your teeth and learn to do it—even at today's prices.

Unfortunately, at the beginning, you have to learn to treat leftover food the way a recently quit smoker treats cigarettes. Many of them boast that they can light up other people's cigarettes, or even let someone blow smoke in their faces. But not until they've quit smoking for a long, long time are they likely to have cigarettes around the house where they might come across them while they're alone. No way. And those ex-smokers who do have cigarettes around are usually called "smokers" again within a short time.

The same is true for leftover food in the refrigerator. You'll probably show marvelous control and self-restraint when others are around, and you may even boast about how you're no longer tempted by things that were once your downfall. But when you're alone, with no one to catch you, things are going to be different. So don't leave goodies around to tempt you in the first place.

That's not to say you should have nothing in your refrigerator. If you do that, you'll only feel sorry for yourself when you open up the door, and that kind of self-pity can lead you to a local take-out place. But only have the right types of foods in there.

If the wrong foods are there, throw them out. Andrea D. finds it easier to throw foods out if she quickly mixes them all together. "Nobody wants to recycle dessert after it's been mixed with the salad and meat," she says. Yuck. A good idea.

ALL AROUND THE HOUSE
A newly thin person is very like a newly dried out

alcoholic. One drink and he's lost again—maybe even forever. You are not exhibiting signs of weakness if you remove temptation from your kitchen shelves, any more than the newly reformed alcoholic is weak when he cleans out his liquor cabinet. You are simply using common sense.

I'm not saying that you can never eat your favorite foods again (although you'd probably be better off if you forgot about cookies and similar sweets and developed a lifelong passion for raw vegetables and such). I am saying that they should not be lying around now to tempt you from the straight and narrow. Keep your refrigerator and your cupboard shelves stocked with those foods that your long years of dieting have taught you are "kosher": raw vegetables, tomato juice, bouillon cubes, water-packed fruit, dry cottage cheese—you know the drill.

Now, say that you've been "just right" for a few weeks and you want to treat yourself to ice cream. You must have ice cream; in fact you can't live without it. O.K. You're a grown-up. Have it—but go out and buy only one portion, not a half gallon. Because if you do the latter, it will then sit in your freezer waiting for—begging for—your next binge. And once it's there, and once you've allowed yourself one dish, why not have two? Why not come back tomorrow and have the rest of it? That stuff is addictive. If you must have a treat now and then, have it, enjoy it, but for God's sake, don't stock up on it.

It also helps to totally eliminate from your home whichever foods were your downfall. For example, if you just couldn't keep your fingers out of a peanut butter jar, banish that wicked substance. Marina S. claims that she hasn't had sugar or salt around for years. "I keep a jar of honey for those occasional too-sour grapefruit halves, or those moments when I just can't stand plain yogurt. And not having salt around keeps me from eating a lot of things I'd be tempted by otherwise. I mean, you've just got to salt leftover steak scraps."

Bread, too, is one substance that may be eliminated completely from your shelves with no ill effects. Nowadays, it's mainly used for holding spreads like butter, margarine and jam, none of which you need anyway, and acting as neat covers for sandwich fillings, which you certainly don't need. If you can't get rid of all of it, though, try what Terry L. did. She could only bring herself to eliminate the outside of her sandwiches. Even so, she was able to cut out many of her lunch calories. Furthermore, rolled-up ham and cheese, speared with a toothpick, has some elegance about it for a lunch.

Other temptations to get rid of in your home are all "decorative" food—bowls of candy, jars of nuts, bowls of raisins, and so on. Recovered alcoholics don't have ice-cold ready-to-drink beer around every ten steps either.

"But what about my family?" you may object. What about your family? Getting rid of items you don't need is not depriving them. You're helping them to learn better eating habits. Do you really want your children to suffer as you have?

Children can buy a treat now and then in the school cafeteria, or from the Good Humor man. Nonaddicted mates can indulge when away from the house. But the whole family will do better on a less rich, less sweet, less accessible diet. And the dental bills will reflect the change too.

KEEP YOUR FOOD PLANNING SIMPLE

Now is not the time to try complicated recipes, particularly those that involve sauces, which are invitations to excessive tasting binges. What happens is that, as Rita L. says, "When I do really fancy cooking, I want to do really fancy eating."

But eating wisely doesn't mean you have to deny yourself a full good-tasting nourishing meal. Instead of pâté, the appetizer can be a raw vegetable, perhaps with a yogurt dip. (In fact, prepared onion soup mix with yogurt instead of sour cream is much better. Honest.)

If you're a soup lover, be careful with the soup you choose. Golden with fat or cream, or heavy with vegetables that have had the nutrients cooked out of them—and the fat soaked into them—and then thickened with flour, noodles or rice, most soups do absolutely nothing for the dieter but give him heartburn. A clear consommé, perhaps garnished with some chopped mushrooms or scallions, is a pleasant, low-calorie way to begin a meal. But read the labels. Some canned broth is not as good a buy, in terms of calories, as bouillon cubes.

When it comes to the main dish, most dieters do well on simple, high protein foods. Chicken, fish,

222

and lean meat are dinner staples, but look for recipes that don't call for frying, added fat, starches, sweetening, or sauces.

If you get a lot of flack from your family and friends about "plain cooking made still plainer by plain cooks," take it in your stride. Sure, your home environment is going to seem rather dull for a while, compared with a gourmet restaurant or even a fast-food emporium. It's the only way, though.

Simplify. Sauces and gravies, for instance, are a particular booby trap for those who must watch their weight. They add little nutritional value, don't make a meal more filling, and can as much as double its calorie content. And if they're made with butter, or derive their richness from fat rendered from the meat while it's cooking, they also add unneeded cholesterol.

That doesn't mean that food has to be dry, though. Most meat (and poultry) has enough internal fat to moisten it. A little dry white wine, tomato juice, lemon juice, or broth can be added where appropriate.

For vegetables (and salads), stick to low-calorie, low-carbohydrate standbys, like lettuce, tomatoes, celery, cucumbers, brussels sprouts, cauliflower, etc. Spinach, zucchini, and cauliflower, for example, are delicious raw, perhaps with a low-calorie dressing or just plain lemon juice. And that famous tomato can be halved and broiled, with a sprinkling of garlic, basil, and oregano.

The intelligent dieter will have his or her favorite piquant spices and seasoning on hand at all times. In addition, capers, horseradish, hot mustard, hot peppers, are all good examples of high-taste, low quantity "necessities" to dieters whose taste buds get a feeling of deprivation without them. An olive or two can satisfy a craving—but be careful. As with pickles: limit yourself.

And dessert doesn't have to be your downfall anymore. Many people just don't feel a meal is over until they have dessert. Fine, finish your meal with one. How about fruit? It provides a recognizable end to a meal—the sweet taste we've all come to expect—with relatively few calories and a great deal of food value. That is, provided that it hasn't been prepared with added sugar, or that you don't overdo it.

In fact, some vitamin researchers suspect that the craving for sweets is a misreading of the body's craving for Vitamin C. So when we think we want a candy bar, we may really want something like an orange. Try fruits high in Vitamin C for dessert; you may find that they supply all the "sweetness" you think you want.

My own favorite is a baked apple. It's not necessary to add sugar to baking apples; simply sprinkle them with cinnamon, nutmeg, and lemon juice—and bake. The same basic recipe can be used on other fruits—pears, for instance—and there's nothing quite as delicious as a grapefruit half gently spiced and run under the broiler.

Later on, you'll be able to live in a kitchen stacked with chocolate bits (in case someone wants to make cookies), just as the reformed alcoholic eventually learns to keep his liquor cabinet stocked so he can serve drinks to other people. But for now, banish temptation from your door and enlist the aid of your family, friends, and guests to keep it that way.

Your home should be your haven—the place where you shed the tensions of the day, relax, and feel comfortable. If you have to walk through your kitchen as if it were a minefield, gritting your teeth and clenching your fists to keep from opening the cupboard or the refrigerator and finding mouth-watering snacks lurking inside, you're putting yourself under unnecessary and undesirable stress.

Control your home environment. Strip it of temptations and fattening foods, and keep it stocked with items that will help you with your diet, not hinder it. A man's home is indeed his castle, but make sure yours isn't a gingerbread house or a candy palace.

13
Shopping Thin

You're at the stage now where the generalities of the Stay Thin program are familiar to you, and you have a good grasp of your individual Stay Thin program. You've learned a lot about eating-behavior at home and at the office and with an occasional minor lapse you're probably able to cope pretty well in those places.

Now it's time to sally forth, to put yourself in situations of risk. These next chapters will deal with these situations—the supermarket, travel, restaurants, resorts and hotels, and, that most risky situation of all—other people. Just as it's easier to diet when you're alone, and when your eating plan is rigid and circumscribed, it's harder to resist temptation when you're preoccupied with other things and other people. Someone will pass a tray of goodies, and you'll take seven before you realize you've taken even one. These tough situations will crop up, and you need to have adequate defense tactics.

Your first hurdle—and it's a biggie—is the supermarket. How you buy—when, how much, what—will dramatically influence what you eat. Once you've committed yourself to buying a bag of celery, you'll probably *eat* celery. Great. Once you've decided to buy a bag of potato chips, you'll no doubt consume that. Not so great. Only you can decide whether or not to hunker down in front of the television set with that bowl of potato chips (which you probably bought) or the celery. And that choice begins in the supermarket aisle. And making those choices when you shop makes it infinitely easier to stick to your guns when you prepare your food and eat it.

Before food goes into your mouth, into your stomach, and unfortunately onto your hips, it has to get into your kitchen. The supermarket manager will never try to persuade you to buy cake, candy and pretzels. He's probably happer if you fill your shopping cart with fresh fruits, vegetables and lean meats. Those items cost more. But the supermarket is arranged according to the food buying habits of most Americans, and we all know that those habits are mostly wrong responses. The aisles of the supermarket feature junk foods often in large colorful packages, with bargains galore, free coupons, and all sorts of other gimmicks to waylay the unwary.

So let's take a long hard look at your supermarket habits and see if we can come up with some guidelines for improving them.

STOP RELYING ON INSTINCT

"I can do it with my eyes closed," says a veteran shopper. She probably does, and you probably do, too. Most of us don't really think when we shop; we are programmed. And our instincts about food are not very sound. Long years of self-destructive overeating have warped those instincts so that they no longer work in our favor. Just as our instincts prompt us to eat too much of the wrong foods, they prompt us to buy the wrong foods to begin with.

Our buying patterns have been programmed by television advertising (notice how the shopping carts in commercials are always overloaded?), by magazine and newspaper advertising, and by life itself. Observe your fellow shoppers on your next marketing trip. Watch what they buy. Economical? Hardly. Fattening? You bet.

Your job now is to reeducate those over-programmed instincts. Start by analyzing your shopping habits.

Let's begin with your list. Do you keep one? Do you follow it? Most of us use a combination of habit, memory, and impulse when we go to the market. Our actual written list, if we use one, is likely to consist mainly of easily forgettable (and nonfattening) items that might not catch our eye or our attention: sixty-watt bulbs, kitty litter, cream of tartar. Few fatties include an item like corn chips on their list. Who needs to? That is the thing that finds its way into our shopping carts through instinct and impulse, a momentary glance, a pang of craving or false hunger.

As an exercise, for the next few weeks make a list every time you go to a market, and try to buy only what is on the list. Discipline like this would never work on a long-term basis, but is good as a kind of consciousness-raising device to help make you more aware of the difference between what you need and what you buy on impulse.

Watch and analyze your pattern of impulse buying. Are you a Collector? A Squirrel? A Sampler? A Hoarder? *Don't* buy food with the indefinite future in mind. Buy only what you need now. And remember that herbs and spices have a limited life span, so while "being prepared" may work fine for a scout, it probably won't for you.

In fact, being a collector in general can be dangerous. Thelma K. was a "what-if" collector: what if ten people suddenly come for cocktails? What if that new man decides to stay for dinner or, hopefully, even for breakfast? Yes, but what if he doesn't? Then, Thelma would eat up all the stuff she'd bought "just in case" to make sure it didn't go to waste.

Which reminds me of Aunt Shirley, who began her career as a housewife during World War II, when food was rationed. Shirley is a Squirrel. Instead of buying one jar of pickles, she buys a dozen. "You never can tell," she says, "they might get scarce." It hasn't happened so far, but she ends up eating pickles with every meal in order to use them up. She is not a thin lady.

Sampling is another trap. Some shoppers are simply fascinated every time they see a new product, or even an old one dressed in a new package. Baby carrots in lemon sauce? Mmmm, must try that. Peanut-butter corn-flakes? Sounds interesting. And, being thrifty-minded, once a shopper has bought this item, she (he) usually feels compelled to use it up, thus paving the way to Lane Bryant.

A word of warning here: children are inveterate samplers, and they don't worry about either weight or their pocketbooks. They just react to packaging, merchandising, and the call of their ever empty little stomachs. Thus, they ask for everything they see. So try not to take them with you to the market. But if you must, train them early in the ways of Stay Thin shopping; explain—and be firm about it—that you're there to buy only what's on your list.

A good list, carefully followed, will help you avoid impulse buying. It will tell you a lot about your food-buying habits. So break down your list resistance. Mary S. was determined to go shopping without a list. When I asked her how she knew what to buy, she replied, "I don't need to make a list. Just seeing something on the shelf reminds me that I need it. And I have a good memory anyway."

We discovered, when I had bullied her into preparing her first lists, and we analyzed them together, that her weekly grocery bill was 40 percent higher than it should have been. But worse, in order to justify her spending, she was eating the extra food items she had not needed in the first place. Just like Aunt Shirley and her pickles.

If you get a mental block or a writer's cramp the

first time you try to make a list, here's a piece of reverse strategy you can use a couple of times. When you come home from the market, make a list of what you've bought—everything. Analyze it. Have you collected, squirreled, or sampled? Have you relied on instinct or impulse? Have you bought items in response to TV commercials rather than your needs? Or have you truly planned and bought only what you need? From those things you bought and need, and those you realize you didn't need, outline your shopping list for the next week.

BEGIN BY TAKING INVENTORY

Here's an excellent opportunity to clean out your kitchen shelves and cabinets. Hell, why not make a day of it. Take everything out. You'll find lots of surprises and not all of them pleasant: last Easter's food coloring, with the lid off; a moldy box of corn-muffin mix; some fossilized raisins. We all have these little skeletons in our kitchen cabinets and every once in a while, all our ghosts must be exorcized.

Do it today. Get inspired. Spray and clean the interior of your cabinets; put down fresh shelf paper; stand back and survey your work. Aren't you wonderful? Surely you don't ever want to put anything unnecessary, gross, or fattening back in there, do you?

Now, turn your attention to the items you have removed from those shelves. The next part is the hardest, particularly for Squirrels. **Discard.** Or as they say in tennis, when in doubt, let it out. You know what your dieting needs and restrictions are: follow them. Throw out not only stuff that's stale and half used up and ancient anyway; also throw out the stuff that has no nutritional value, or that might tempt you on a binge. Connie S. did this the other day. "It showed me a lot about the kinds of things I tend to snack on—half used-up packages of chocolate bits, raisins out of the box, dried cold cereals. The clean-up job helped me make a resolution: I'm starting fresh."

Now, organize those shelves you've just cleaned out. Place all remaining items so that you can see them. This will help you avoid buying baking soda over and over again, and ending up with four boxes. If it's only baking soda, it's no real problem. But what if it's chocolate bits?

Now look at what's left. In taking a food inventory, there are a few things to keep in mind.

1. Don't take inventory on an empty stomach (and don't shop on one either—but everyone knows that).

2. Don't be afraid to cut your losses. Junk food? Throw it out. Sweet treats? Get rid of them. The money you throw away doing this will be saved later since Staying Thin is cheaper than being fat.

3. Try to figure out what you don't have. Maybe there are items you've been forgetting for years: good herbs, an extra jar of diet mayonnaise. These are positive items.

4. Work out a new system of organization. Janet keeps everything in alphabetical order, so

that it's easy to run her eye along the shelf and see what needs replenishing. Marlene L. finds that system stultifying. She keeps a small pad of paper and a pencil next to the food cupboard, and simply writes down the items when she throws away the last box.

And while you're at it, take a nonfood inventory to make sure you're well stocked. Why mention this in a food-related book? Because you want to limit your trips to the market as much as possible, and often those trips are triggered by the need for a bottle of window-washing fluid or some furniture polish. Every time you enter the supermarket to buy some soap pads, toothpaste, or paper towels, you put yourself in the path of temptation.

The more time you spend in the supermarket, the more likely you are to buy food—and naturally to eat it. Every trip you make there should be a no-frills business venture. So if you become aware (and keep a list to remind you) of the items that usually reside in the bathroom closet, under the sink, and in the cleaning cabinet, you'll be doing yourself a big favor.

To return to your list, plan it to get you out of the market fast. Time is not only money (you'll spend) but food (you'll eat). Market researchers have calculated to the penny how much money people spend with each extra minute in the market. If supermarkets had to rely on people who bought only what they needed, they would go out of business.

But if you're like most people, you shop like a yo-yo, bouncing back and forth between the aisles as you grab both the items from the list and the ones your impulses suggest. You keep back-tracking and recovering the same areas, making it more likely you will buy the items you may have wisely resisted the first time around.

Instead, think of yourself as an efficiency expert, and figure out how to do the most work in the least time. Before you leave your house, or as you're planning your list, picture your store—you can even sketch a diagram if that makes it easier. Write down each item in the order you will pick it up as you move through the aisles. Plan to go down each aisle only once, using the shortest, most direct route through the store.

Learn the overall plan of your market, and follow the same route each time. Learn the pitfalls also—your individual ones—in your market. Which aisle contains the most temptations? Where do you linger longest? Which items are hardest to resist? Knowing your weaknesses is half the battle.

Here are a few other tips about supermarket shopping, some of which you've heard before; unfortunately, probably none of which you've followed before. Make it different this time.

1. Just as you shouldn't prepare your shopping list when you're hungry, you should never go into a supermarket when you're ready for a meal. Many people find that supermarkets are emptiest in the mornings; try shopping after a nice solid breakfast. Chances are fewer goodies will appeal

to you at that hour of the day.

2. Don't be obsessed with looking for bargains. The effort to Stay Thin may entail a little more in the way of expenditure at first, and a little less in the way of bargain hunting, since the bargains are usually fattening items. So what if you have a coupon for potato chips? Throw it away or give it to a thin friend. If an item is not on your list, don't buy it, no matter how cheap it is. Save your bargain-hunting instincts for non-food items like cat food, detergent, or a case of paper towels which won't put an extra inch on your middle.

3. Don't touch food items. Studies have shown that once you touch an item, you're much more likely to buy it than if you just stood there and stared at it. Supermarket managers know this, and that's why higher-priced items are often placed in prominent positions. If you think you're about to touch an item, just say to yourself, "If I touch it, I'll probably buy it; if I buy it, I'll most likely eat it; if I eat it, I'll definitely get fat again."

4. Beware of the front of the supermarket and the checkout line. While the entire market is a seductive trap, the front part, usually where the checking line is, is the most enticing of all. Your guard is down. You're standing around, waiting. As you wait for the person in front of you to empty his or her basket, or as the checker pauses to put another roll of paper in the cash register, your eye is caught by those convenient small candy rolls, cookie specials, and other fattening items. Pick up a magazine or newspaper instead. Junk reading carries fewer penalties than junk food.

5. As I mentioned earlier, learn to shop less often. Study your shopping habits. How often are you going to the market? Do you do one major weekly trip and then stop by and "pick up a few things" every day or so? These casual trips—intended to pick up an extra quart of milk or some forgotten item—are often dangerous. Try to cut down on them. Make your list so superefficient that you don't need those side trips any more.

6. Edit your list before you leave. Go over it carefully and cross out any items you don't really need, especially those that will interfere with your diet.

7. Confine your shopping to one store. Whatever you do, don't let impulse buying strike when you're off your guard—say in the gourmet department of your favorite department store, or in that cute little dried-fruit-and-nut shop just as you get off the bus. When you're shopping, shop. The rest of the time, resist.

Like any other activity—skiing, tennis, driving a car—you'll derive more pleasure and satisfaction from shopping if you do it well. Observe your fellow man, and woman, in your supermarket. Look at those confused, befuddled expressions. Watch the way some people scuttle from aisle to aisle like frenzied chickens. Listen to those deep sighs, observe those frowns, watch those hesitating fingers as someone ruminates endlessly over which can of tuna fish to buy.

Efficient shopping is liberating. You'll get out of there in less time with less stress and strain, and you'll have the good feeling of a job well done.

Happy list-making, happy marketing—and don't forget the cottage cheese.

14
Traveling Thin:
Eating Away From Home

If you never had to go anyplace except your home, your job, and your supermarket, you *might* be temptation-free, and able to cope effortlessly with your Stay Thin regime. But you *do* go other places, you do encounter other people (some of them maddeningly thin), and you do get caught in unexpected situations.

So let's make another list. This time, try lists of all the situations, away from home, that have caused you to pig out in the past. List the people you know (maybe a friend who always prepares rich desserts and talks you into eating them, for instance) who tend to trigger food binges. People, places, situations—list them all.

Some of my patients made lists like these in a recent evening class. Ginger P., whose husband travels a lot but is one of the dying breed who won't ride in airplanes, goes on many ocean voyages. So she put cruises on the top of her list.

"You live from meal to meal on a ship," Ginger says. "Enormous breakfasts, a snack at eleven, a gigantic lunch, then a nap, teatime, and a dinner that goes on all evening until the midnight buffet. And in between, you don't do much but maybe play a little shuffleboard. I just *can't* keep my weight down on those trips."

Nathan P., a handsome but potbellied young bachelor, has problems with a different kind of boat—his sailboat. "We go out for the day, drink beer, eat snacks, then put into port and have a huge lobster dinner. That salt air makes me ravenous."

Paula S. blames her downfall on summer vacations at a mountain resort. "Three big meals a day, and no cooking, shopping, or cleaning up. I just revel in it. And the food is so *rich.* Do you know, one summer the kids made a bet with each other that they would have something *à la mode* every day for dessert at *both* lunch and dinner—and they did it!"

For Paul de A., a magazine editor, the problem is business lunches. He's under a lot of pressure to find and commission the most up-to-date and exciting articles, and he must woo authors fairly lavishly. "I take them to a good restaurant, we have a few drinks, and my mind is on making a deal. If you asked me afterwards what I'd had to eat, all you'd get is a blank look. But I know that those lunches really put on the pounds—my scales tell me so."

239

And for Norma G., her nemesis is the apartment of her best friend, Ginny. Ginny is skinny—in fact, she has always been known as "skinny Ginny." And she's also a real pig. From the moment Norma walks in the door, she is bombarded with treats—Ginny's homemade ice cream, Ginny's cookies, Ginny's chocolate cake. "We get to talking, and the afternoon just flies. So does my resolve not to eat. I do it without even *noticing*. I never snack when I'm at home. Only at Ginny's."

Obviously, what everyone needs is a method for dealing with such contingencies. Like a general planning a battle, you've got to figure out every direction the enemy could be coming from, every move he might make. You must anticipate every trick, and be ready to counter each sneak attack—or rather snack attack—with every possible kind of offensive and defensive strategy.

THE SECRET IS PLANNING

It is not within the scope of this book to tell you what diet to go on, or how to diet. That's between you and your doctor, or you and your common sense. But regardless of what you're eating, there's one crucial ingredient when it comes to Staying Thin. Planning.

Throughout this book we've talked about planning alternate responses to food-provoking situations: planning conditions in your home, planning the kinds of food you eat and even planning how to buy it. If you do these things haphazardly, dealing with them only when they come up, the effect

240

will be hazardous to your dietary health.

But up to this point we've been talking about things *you* can control—your free time, your home, your shopping list. It's a little harder to plan things when you're not the one in charge, when someone else does the shopping, the cooking, and the serving. Since you've relinquished control of all aspects of food preparation, it's natural to let go of your self-control as well. Isn't it true that when you go away on vacation you eat as much in a week as a family of four would? Because you paid for it, because someone else did all the hard work, because others are eating, because you want to enjoy yourself, because you're on vacation, because it's there—

But the truth is that nothing is any different—about your weight, anyway—just because you're away from home. Pasta, bread, and ice cream sundaes contain just as many calories, and will add as many extra pounds in Shangri-La as they will in suburbia. So, just because you plan to be away, whether just out to lunch, at a dinner party, or on a world cruise, don't stop planning to lose weight and Stay Thin.

HOW TO PLAN RESTAURANT MEALS

Let's start with the most common away-from-home pitfall: the restaurant. Everybody ends up in restaurants from time to time. Some on a daily basis. Others perhaps only during one continuous two-week binge on a resort vacation. But whatever your situation, however often it happens, the rules are basically the same. And most find them difficult.

But David M. thinks that dining in a restaurant is actually easier on his diet than any other kind of eating. For one thing, once his portion is finished, he can't have seconds. "Unless I'm willing to pay and wait for them," he notes, "which I'm not." Also, his waiter does not really push more food at him ("unlike my wife") beyond simply asking, "Will there be any anything else?" And it gives him a chance to have foods he loves and can't resist—but under circumstances in which portions are controlled.

But a restaurant, just like a kitchen, can be a tempting trap for many dieters. Restaurant food, for example, is more carefully arranged than most home-cooked food, and is therefore more visually appealing. And when dieters see what others are getting, carried tantalizingly above the tables, even the most determined Stay Thinner may waver.

So it's good to be aware that you'll be tempted, and plan ways to resist before you even open the restaurant door:

1. Choose an appropriate restaurant in the first place. Why patronize eateries with names like "The Pasta Factory," or "Ye Old Sweete Shoppe"? That's asking for trouble. Where then should you eat? Let me tell you about John T.'s experience.

John, a businessman who, like Paul, must wine and dine clients, finds it excruciatingly difficult to resist temptation. "When I take a client out to lunch, he usually takes advantage of my expense account," John says. "He orders two or three drinks and the kind of food his doctor—and mine—has ordered him to stay away from. You know—steak, whipped cream with dessert, the works. And I have to take him to a *good* restaurant, so the stuff looks even more gorgeous than it must taste. The guy looks so damn happy eating it, it's more than I can stand."

John was able to eliminate some of the temptations of entertaining clients simply by changing the kind of restaurant he takes them to. Now they dine at Japanese or Chinese restaurants where desserts don't loom large on the menu. Nor is bread served at the table.

Also, oriental food, not prepared with animal fats, and frequently cooked with large amounts of low carbohydrate vegetables, is generally lower in cholesterol and calories than most standard restaurant fare. Another plus: in most Chinese restaurants, the serving dishes generally have covers shielding the dieter from the tempting sight of someone else's delicacies. If the client balks at oriental food, John takes him to a seafood restaurant, where the client can have his "surf and turf" while John enjoys filet of lemon sole.

2. It helps to write your choices down. Just as you're more likely to keep to a written shopping list, you're more likely to keep to a written menu order.

3. Remember that alcoholic beverages are high in calories while providing practically zip in nutrition. If you feel you must drink, choose white

wine at seventy-five calories for about three ounces. That's a better choice than Scotch at two hundred fifty calories for the same amount. And you'll get less loaded—and therefore weaker—too.

Drinking in public has become easier for dieters now that sparkling waters are fashionable. "A glass of Perrier water and a squeeze of lime makes me look with it these days, not like a wet blanket," John reports. "Also, I'm better able to do business without three martinis under my belt." And they definitely *were* under his belt.

4. From now on, plan to order all meals *à la carte*. Few people, whether or not they're watching their weight, can turn down food they feel is free or already paid for. You're far more likely to pass up dessert if you have to pay extra for it than if it comes with the meal. Ditto for appetizer, soup, rolls and salad layered with creamy dressing.

5. Realize that the salad bar is not for you. The salad bar is a hot new gimmick in restaurants today. Customers like it because it's fun to pick and choose. But for a dieter, that kind of fun is skating on thin ice. Sure, there're lettuce, cucumbers, tomatoes, onions. But there're also bacon, cheeses, dressings (oozing with oil), croutons, bread and butter, pickles and (as they say in the ads), much, much more.

Also, it's so easy to load your plate, and come back for seconds and even thirds, telling yourself all the while "it's only salad. It's low-calorie. It's good for me, and if I fill up on that, I won't go overboard with the high-calorie hamburger." Yes, but a salad with all the junk on it can easily come to 600 calories, while a three-four ounce hamburger is only around 400.

It's far safer, if you hunger for a salad, to plan to order one with your meal, dressed only with lemon juice or vinegar. Or bring your own low-calorie dressing in one of those little plastic bottles you can buy at the five and ten. Sure, it may look a bit strange when you take the bottle out of your purse and pour the liquid on your salad, but don't worry about it.

6. Be assertive. You're overpaying for the food as it is. If you feel badly about asking them to do something special for you, you can leave an extra tip. Get it through your head that you've worked hard on this weight thing, and you don't have to eat what you don't want to eat.

One of my former patients, who has kept her weight down for over a year, had a good solution to the recalcitrant waiter problem. She tells him she's allergic to butter, salad dressing, hollandaise sauce on the asparagus, whatever, rather than simply asking him to omit it. Somehow, this compelling medical reason makes more of an impression, perhaps because the restaurant is afraid of being held liable if she really is telling the truth.

7. If you really want that small portion, you

might try ordering a child's plate. Not all restaurants will serve a child's portion to an adult, so it's best to inquire ahead of time, by telephone. The phone, by the way, will shield you from disquieting looks.

8. If possible, plan to bring along just enough money to pay for the type of *à la carte* meal you've decided on. That might keep you from ordering more than you had planned. If you've got an expense account, then try pretending, like our businessman John T. does, that your expense account doesn't cover dessert. Then, it's less of a fait accompli that he'll order it.

What if someone else is taking you out on his or her expense account? There's no easy way around this. We all like the feeling of having a little luxury for nothing. So the best way is to pretend you're paying for it yourself. Again, set a limit—a moderate one—and stay with it.

9. Arrange to share your restaurant expedition with a sympathetic dinner companion. It's not much fun to sit opposite someone gleefully packing away all your favorite foods and then ordering seconds of them. And if that person knows you're trying to keep your weight down, and teases you about it, your resolve may be undermined, or indeed your evening totally demolished. It helps if your nearest companion knows your secret and gives you support, even the unspoken kind.

10. Don't forget your Stay Thin techniques. You don't leave your good manners behind when

you dine out, so why should you abandon your Stay Thin techniques? Remember, eat slowly, in small mouthfuls; concentrate on chewing and tasting (no matter how pleasant the company), and stop when—or before—you feel full. Just as at home, you may do best by filling up on the lower-calorie portions of your meal, such as your salad, first.

Or you might follow the lead of Dottie P., who lost thirty-five pounds and has kept them off for three years.

When Dottie went to restaurants and found all that food on her plate, she would heavily pepper those parts of each dish she felt she should do without. Since using pepper looks natural enough, no one with her realized she was deliberately trying to spoil her food.

If overpeppering sounds too drastic to you—or if you're an ardent pepper-lover—try a little rearranging. For example, put the bread tray on the far end of the table, or ask the waiter to remove it altogether. Shirley Z., a social worker, reports great success in forgetting about the bread by casually draping a napkin over it as if she was trying to keep it warm.

One Stay Thin technique does not apply to eating out: while you may want the meal to last a long time, that's certainly not true of the dessert course. If your companions are lingering over their luscious desserts and coffee, get up and go make some phone calls. Some people do this to pretend they're more important than they are; and you have an even better reason.

11. If possible, plan an activity after the meal. If you go directly home, especially when you're alone, you may be tempted to extend the festive feeling by eating more. And why not? You behaved in the restaurant. Surely you deserve a reward? So, go to a movie, or for a walk—and *then* go home.

Although I've stressed its negative aspects, dining out, once you know the ropes, is good for the soul. You change the scenery, someone else handles all the details of food preparation (within your requirements), you feel festive, you have fun. People need fun, especially if they're giving up pleasures they've been used to. An unexpected plus is that you dress up for a special meal out. If your weight is consistently going down, you can see yourself looking better and better, and this helps reinforce your determination.

OTHER PEOPLE'S HOUSES— ## ANOTHER TRAP

Another tough situation—often more difficult than restaurant dining—is socializing in other people's homes. Here, you run the added risk of insulting people if you don't sample the party food they've prepared, and you're much less in control of what you eat than you are in a restaurant. If Cousin Hattie serves spaghetti, you can't quietly order broiled fish, hold the butter, instead.

The Golden Rule for Stay Thin eating in company is simply this: Be up front about it. Let people know you are dieting. Tell them firmly, and quietly, and then shut up. (Nobody wants to hear your calorie count or your poundage details.)

It used to be considered rude to eat differently from other guests at a party, but the rules have changed, partly, because we have added awareness of health today. In fact, people who don't drink often go to parties armed with a bottle of Perrier water or a container of sugar-free iced-tea mix. So if your diet is a rigid one, take your water-pack tuna along in a plastic bag. But do inform your hostess ahead of time; otherwise, it *is* rude.

Dinner parties—especially the sit-down kind, where you're likely to spend the whole evening at the table—are the toughest. Cocktail parties, buffets, coffee klatches, even wedding receptions are easier, because you move around a lot and nobody pays much attention to what anyone else is eating, or if, in fact, you are eating.

One of the problems with dinner parties is that it's a rare host or hostess who'll discuss his or her menu in advance, and an even rarer one who doesn't want to impress with his or her culinary expertise by serving a knockout, heavily sauced, several-course dinner.

If you're not sure that you're going to find yourself in safe territory, call your host or hostess beforehand and explain your situation. And while you're on the phone, offer to bring the dessert. This will pacify the cook and give you some measure of control over the meal. Is there some dessert you hate? Sy G. hates buttercream frosting—it's so rich it makes him gag—but he's a sucker for real whipped cream. Do you think he brings along strawberry shortcake? No. Lemon—his most hated flavor—buttercream.

One of the hazards of social eating is that in the sheer pleasure of other people's company or even one person's company you are hardly aware that you're eating the whole thing. Even in the most casual social situation, say with just one friend at an afternoon coffee klatsch in the kitchen (aha!), your inhibitions and your will power disappear.

For example, Max and Janie, a happily married couple for seven years, put on over 100 pounds together just sitting in the kitchen when Max came home, talking about the day's events while Janie was preparing dinner. But as they chatted, they nibbled on crackers, pretzels, cheese, whatever else was at hand, not to mention having a couple of before-dinner drinks each.

The solution: they ultimately formed the new habit of communicating with each other when food was *not* present. Or of saving up their small talk for dinner, when they were eating what they had planned to eat, not impulse items.

Arthur S. decided that he didn't want to give up the wonderful combination of food and talk he enjoyed with his friends at his girlfriend Margie's apartment, but he didn't want to get fat either. Now, along with the wine, he brings a gift of a platter of raw vegetables to be served with the other hors d'oeuvres. "I find Marge is delighted to have an extra dish," he reports, "but there's still a problem. Everybody else gets to the low-calorie tray first!'' Indeed, so many people are watching their weight nowadays that a savvy host or hostess will be a success if he or she serves an interesting assortment of low-calorie goodies without waiting for an Arthur to bring them.

Barbara M. has found her own way to handle social occasions that might lead to a diet downfall. She wears a special ring she calls her ''fat ring'' to such events. A few years ago, when she weighed forty pounds more than she does today, she was unable to take that ring off her finger. Finally, she had to undergo the discomfort (not to mention the humiliation) of having the ring cut off.

Now, at a party, one glance at that hand fetching food to her mouth is enough to make her put the food down. ''I never want to be that way again,'' she says. ''Never, never, never. And the ring reminds me, in case I forget, how I got to be so fat in the first place.''

You may have some small, hardly noticeable item that can stiffen your resolve at parties. Maybe it's something to wear, like a skirt that feels tight around your hips the moment you gain a pound. It doesn't even have to have any associations with your weight. You might tell yourself, for example, that whenever you put your hand in your pocket and touch a Kennedy half-dollar you can always carry, you'll remember to go easy on the snack tray.

Or you might try Raymond W.'s example. He does well at dinner parties except for the hors d'oeuvres and dessert. Naturally. So now he arrives fashionably late (having filled himself up at home on bouillon), and misses those tempting little platters of tidbits and the second or third round of drinks as well. Later when the dessert course is served, he manages to find himself a book, in his host's library. At one home where he goes frequently, he instead offers to walk the dog. "There goes Raymond," his friends say. They laugh about it—and so does Raymond—but they understand his problem and respect his ability to cope with it.

Margot E. psychs herself out of wanting dessert. "I tell myself it's filled with poison, like the cake in *Peter Pan*. And it really *is*—poison to the thin me, anyway." This is an example of how the imagination—the "let's pretend" that all of us have hidden within us—can help in diet situations. Pretend it's poisoned. Pretend it's spoiled and yucky. Pretend it will make you break out in hives. (But you don't have to pretend that it will make you fat.)

Sometimes, of course, you'll find yourself at a party where none of those hints will work. At convention dinners, or large dinner dances, you may be a captive at the table for hours on end, perhaps while speeches (invariably dull) are being made. Often, at large gatherings like these, your plate is simply placed in front of you, and you are forced to sit—often for a long time—staring at an enormous, fatty slab of roast beef, a baked potato with sour cream, and some watery (no doubt canned) string beans. The salad, if there is one, is usually uncrisp and swimming in fattening dressing. And banquets such as this—and here we can include wedding dinners, bar mitzvahs, all enormous sit-down affairs—*always* seem to feature ice cream or cake for dessert, usually with a sauce.

You may, on these occasions, simply have to bite the bullet. Or the meat. Take a few bites of the meat, and *hope* that your dinner companion, or the speaker, is interesting enough to steer your attention away from the food. If there's dancing, dance every dance.

Each of you, I'm sure, has some other social event that's particularly hard on your dieting. "Pot luck" church suppers, Girl Scout picnics, company outings, family reunions, all are fraught with peril. Awareness of the dangers, as always, is a giant step toward restraint.

By now, it may sound as if all the booby traps are found in restaurants, hotel ballrooms, and other people's houses. But the same things can happen when you give a party. Just because you stick to Stay Thin Perrier water, doesn't mean you expect your guests to do the same; you'll have to offer a selection of drinks. And you can't serve only broiled fish and salad at a dinner party. So, you'll have to face (and prepare) a lot of foods that you're not going to eat yourself—and you can't arrive late. But you can prepare your own raw vegetable dish to munch on while preparing food, and you can fill yourself up with a lot of bouillon beforehand.

Just remember: holidays, vacations, evenings out, and even your own parties are supposed to be fun. And afterwards, you want to be refreshed, rejuvenated, and relaxed—not guilty that you made a pig of yourself. And not any fatter than when you arrived there.

It's a tough balance to strike—but you can do it.

15
Socializing Thin:
Coping With Other People

In an earlier chapter the point was made that drinking and smoking are easier vices to cure than overeating, because you can't give eating up entirely. People can't be given up either. And in some cases, they can be almost as dangerous to you as food.

Therefore, you must develop an awareness of the ways in which other people can—consciously or unconsciously—undermine your dieting resolves, and learn various strategies for dealing with this.

For example, fatness can be used by others as a weapon to make you miserable just as you may be using your weight to be doing this to them. When Cheryl first married, she had been a slim attractive coed. Ten years, and three pregnancies later, she was fifty pounds heavier than she had been as a bride. Her husband's callous friends kidded him about his hefty wife, and he hated to take her out in public, sure that he was being pitied behind his back by friends whose wives were still sexy.

After putting up with endless nagging, she finally managed to shed most of the excess weight. But then, her husband suddenly became alarmed. Not only was his wife glorying in her rediscovered attractiveness, but so were other men. Subconsciously, he began to miss the unattractive but safe woman she'd become.

So he started telling her she was getting so thin she'd get sick, and urging her to eat more. "You went too far," he would tell her. "I like to have some rump to pinch. Forget about all this starvation—it's making you cranky anyway—and put some meat back on your bones." With this kind of "support" and the pressure off—in fact reversed—her resolve evaporated, leaving her diet program a shambles.

Although it may be obvious to others that this kind of behavior is destructive, those involved often sincerely think that they're helping. "I'm only doing it for his (her) own good," they insist.

But a case like this illustrates what we call "sabotage behavior," which can be motivated by many things. A mother can worry about her fourteen-year-old daughter's budding sexuality, and unconsciously try to defuse it by ensuring through the type of meals she serves that her daughter will get fat. Or mother, unconsciously jealous of her son's growing interest in girls, may take the same tack: if he's overweight, she may subconsciously reason, he will have trouble dating.

A daughter who feels guilty about neglecting her mother may even try to force feed her when she comes for Sunday dinner even though the old lady has been trying to keep her weight down for years. Or a well-meaning father who grew up during the Depression may stuff his children so that they "won't have to suffer like I did." Except that, of course, they will often suffer in other ways.

What makes things more complicated is that sometimes subversive behavior is difficult to detect. The way others around you react to your weight loss is rarely a cut and dry, approval or disapproval affair, and often it changes from day to day.

Members of our Stay Thin group identified several types of people whose behavior in the past had affected their diets. You may recognize some of these types from your own experience, and you have others to add to the list.

The Cold Shoulder. These people ignore you anyway, shrug their shoulders, or grunt. It's their approved method of communication in most instances. They don't give you any real feedback—about weight loss or about anything else either. "How am I looking?" you ask. "You always look O.K. to me," comes the automatic reply. You can't expect Cold Shoulders to react in any meaningful manner to your self-improvement.

Hand Clappers. These are people who cheerfully give you positive feedback. Their statements suggest that they're pleased that you're doing well and they always seem to say the type of things that will keep you on the right road. "You look better than ever." "I admire your self-control." "You seem like a different person since you lost all that weight."

But deep down, there may be a nagging suspicion on your part about them. Do they really mean what they say, or is this the type of thing they say to everyone regardless? Have they really observed us, or are they just into saying what they think will please others? Therefore, can we trust their statements?

Hedonists. Hedonists may mean well, but their "happiness-now worry-later or do-whatever-makes-you-feel-good-now" philosophy may be disastrous to your dieting.

For example, it's hard to turn down dessert when you're with someone at a restaurant who says things like "Haven't you punished yourself long enough? Enjoy yourself and eat what pleases you." They may be right in their you-live-only-once philosophy—but do you really want to do it as a fatty?

The Heckler. These people totally undermine you. They never treat your plans seriously and put down your efforts. They taunt you with remarks like "At it again, eh? How long will you Stay Thin this time? When will you just give up?" (Once in a while, though, a heckler can cause positive changes in your behavior by making you decide that you'll show them.)

The Confuser. This is someone who gives conflicting advice. On the one hand, Confusers seem to be reinforcing your weight loss; on the other hand, they do everything in their power to undermine it. A typical example would be a hostess who says, "You look great since you lot all that weight, but you must try my new cheesecake." Or a mother who says, "I admire your self-control, but I'll feel just terrible if you don't have any of my pie after I spent all day baking it."

There are others too, like the Fatalists, who tell you you're destined to stay hefty and it's not worth the effort to fight it, or the Jerk who insists that men like fat women better than thin, etc.

Actually many sabotage statements are based on the fact that other people aren't really listening to what you say, not that they have some reason to undermine you, or that they're just creeps to begin with. Most people are so preoccupied with their own problems and concerns, that they never really turn the full beam of their attention on anyone else unless they hear a real cry for help. And even then, sometimes they only give you half of their attention, a quarter of their concern, and an eighth of their understanding.

Bob M.'s secretary, a young newlywed, was a hot and heavy cook. She made cookies, candies, pastries for her new husband, and brought samples to the office for her boss. Despite his burgeoning paunch, Bob accepted her offerings regularly so as not to hurt her feelings. And instead of saying anything *directly* to her, he simply dropped hints about how he shouldn't be eating all these sweets. The bride-gourmet, equally well-intentioned, but equally insensitive, didn't pick up on the cue, and went on serving the sweets. And he went on eating them until he put on ten pounds that way.

Some people don't *want* to hear you. They want to be praised for their culinary skills more than they want to praise you for your weight loss and the work *that* entails. They know you're trying to maintain your weight—yet they offer you fattening foods. The ways they use to persuade you to eat are as varied as their personalities. Sometimes they literally insist that you eat a particular food ("You must try my new . . ."); other times, they approach you in a subtly enticing manner, calculated to make you feel miserable if you refuse. ("I've worked so hard on this; it would make me feel so good if you tasted it"). In some cases, they are conscious of the significance of what they say; other times, they are totally oblivious clods.

It's hard for us to accept the fact that many people we like—in some cases love—really don't want the best for us. Or don't care. They want us to be fat. Why? There are many reasons for this:

1. They're jealous. You've been able to accomplish what they haven't been able to do.

2. Misery loves company. When they see you happy, then they're left all alone with their problems.

3. Competition. They may be afraid of the physical competition the slim you would give to them. This problem often arises when two

overweight people of the same sex are friends, and one loses weight and the other can't.

Women, when they lose weight and start to look attractive, are especially threatening to other women, including those whom they consider their closest friends. Girlfriends start treating them differently. What used to be a friendly relationship may become a bitterly competitive and hostile one.

4. Fear of losing you. They're afraid of losing you now that you look so much better and are probably glowing with overall confidence too. This is a common problem with members of the opposite sex who find the weight loss of one partner threatening—particularly when both are overweight.

5. They're afraid they'll have fewer things to talk to you about. Do you remember when your conversation centered around food—and the avoidance of food—much of the time? Perhaps that's all you really had in common with them.

6. If you're not fat, they have less reason to use you, abuse you, or put you down. Suddenly, you're far less vulnerable than you were, which may make them feel more vulnerable.

The reasons family and friends may not be happy about your improvement are not limited to the above. And any one person will be sure to have more than one reason. Your job is to try to figure out where they are coming from, reassure them that you're still yourself, and try to make the necessary adjustments that your physical and emotional changes require. But don't jump to conclusions about people. You may be superdefensive at this time and prone to make hasty judgments about who your supporters—and detractors—actually are.

HOW TO HANDLE PEOPLE AND STAY THIN

Whatever their reasons, good or bad, for urging you to eat, you must learn to turn a deaf ear. This is the time when *you* come first, and for the purpose of self-preservation, you must disregard what they say.

If you really want to maintain your weight this time, the answer you must give your friends and your loved ones when they insist that you eat is a big **No**. No matter what they say, you say **No**. The only word in your vocabulary at a time like this is **No**.

It's too bad you can't be subtle; it's too bad you can't explain it all again; but if people refuse to cooperate and to pick up on the cues you feed them, you'll just have to get tough and be blunt. **No**. Don't discuss the matter. If you go on talking about it, they'll find chinks in your argument and your resolve may weaken. You've tried reason; now you must start using verbal muscle.

You may also have to start changing some of your friends. It makes it easier to begin with if you avoid associating with Fat Failures—people who have dieted, constantly, and failed, constantly. Many of these people will go out of their way to make you feel as though you are embarked on a doomed venture at the very time when you need emotional support. These are the folks who, five hundred years ago, would have assured Columbus that the earth was flat.

Besides which, they don't set a very good example for you. They're also the most likely ones, consciously or unconsciously, to try to sabotage your plans. After all, if you succeed this time, and never have to go on a diet again, what company will they share their misery with? Fat Failures will end up depressing and undermining you if they catch you in a bad moment. Avoid 'em.

It is important for you, at this time, to surround yourself with boosters, with people who recognize the importance of your weight control efforts (and of whatever you're doing for yourself that's positive), and who will sincerely offer you encouragement and support as you begin your new life as a reformed foodaholic.

A supportive social environment really does help you in your weight control efforts. And with the exception of the Hand clappers, the types we identified earlier—not to mention other people as well—could undermine your efforts to make your last diet your final diet.

So point out to them all that you need *their* help in maintaining your weight loss. Explain to them exactly what you're doing. Let them see that this is not another diet, but a new way of life. Let them know how important it is to you. Most people, if you take them into your confidence, will at least try to cooperate. Request their assistance and tell them you'd appreciate their not offering you food, not discussing it endlessly in your presence, and also, not being so stingy with their praise.

Of course, it's your job to reward those around you when they do cooperate with your weight-loss efforts and encourage you to continue. If people shell out compliments, for instance, take the time to thank them. Otherwise, you may not receive them again. Be sure to let them know exactly how much their support means to you. They may think of you as "independent," so much so that you don't need others to give you moral support. So declare your needs.

As for making new friends, don't let that lead you into going off your diet. Mary S. had just moved into a new singles complex in Texas and didn't know anyone. Meeting men was the easy part, but she kept hoping to make some women friends, too. Any time one of them approached her, however, it was always with a suggestion to go to a restaurant, try some of their homemade ice cream, or come over for a few drinks. Mary kept refusing, because her food-resistance was low, but she realized that she'd never make friends unless she started accepting invitations.

"The next time someone asked me," Mary said, "I told them 'wait till I go back to my apartment and get some diet soda. It's all I can have until dinner.' And, do you know, the girl who was inviting me was pleased with that. She confessed that she felt she had to offer rich food and drink for company—and she didn't even like the stuff.'

Your ability to withstand temptation, particularly under social pressure, will be constantly tested. Another way to prepare for these types of stress is to arm yourself beforehand. Knowing that these tests will arise, rehearse your reponse to them, in front of a mirror if necessary. This way, you will know immediately how to deal with them, rather than stumbling through an improvised excuse.

Let's take a very common example. You are going to be staying with your parents for a period of a few days. You are looking forward to the visit—except for one gnawing problem. Your mother will tempt you constantly with every variety of forbidden pleasure. She'll dangle before you all manner of ice cream, cookies, homemade cakes. She'll make you feel guilty if you don't eat what she "slaved all day over the stove to make." She'll seem hurt, to say the least, if you refuse. How will you handle it?

What you do is practice a little assertiveness in a dry-run no-food setting. Construct a firm but polite rejection. Make it perfectly clear that you would love to indulge, but that it's more important for you to be very careful of your weight at this time. Go over the exact words you will use—and her inevitable argument, which by now you surely know by heart. Say these words over and over until you know them all by heart, and you have your part down pat. Alone, in front of a mirror, you can even rehearse this speech as if you were an actor; hell, you are an actor.

But if this fails the first few times, or you're not assertive enough ever to be able to say no, or maybe the other person is so callous that they just plop the food on your plate anyway, all is still not lost. On your plate doesn't have to mean in your mouth. Cut it up, push it around the plate, and when they tell you that "you haven't touched a thing," insist you have. They're not going to count the morsels that are left over. (If you want to learn how to fake eating food, watch a skinny person eat. "Barely touching their food," is incorrect. They do keep touching it with their fork—to break it up and push it around and pile other foods on top of it. They touch it; they just don't eat it.)

Even when people are not offering you food, you'll probably find it very supportive to tell them how well you're finally doing on your weight maintenance. You'll get praise from those who know and love you, which will help make the difficult moments worthwhile. Don't feel bad about fishing for compliments—and enjoy them when they come along.

But don't overdo. Eating food, and dieting are boring, boring, boring subjects, and nobody can stand to talk about them for very long—except a dieter. Just as a young mother can talk endlessly about diapers and formulas, and a law student can talk endlessly about torts, most dieters talk endlessly about weight and calories—and lose more friends than pounds in the bargain.

It's also important, although not imperative, to try to get your whole family's aid. You can make all the physical changes in your house you can think of, and have all kinds of elaborate plans to avoid snacking while watching TV, phoning, etc., but if everyone around you is eating potato chips and then passing you the bowl, you have a hard row to hoe.

Some families unconsciously try to sabotage the dieting members because dieters really do make those around them miserable; they constantly talk about their diet; sigh and look sad when someone else enjoys a bite of food; piss and moan when they gain an ounce, overdo the joy bit when they lose, etc. This stuff gets boring and some of your family's antagonism in the past may have been justified. Sure, families are supposed to be sympathetic, but they're only human. And sometimes they just get fed up, and understandably try to short-circuit your bitchiness by undermining your diet.

It might (and then, again, it might not) help to explain to your family that this is not a diet. You're not going to starve yourself and become bitchy again. You are just going to change some of the cues associated with eating, so that you *never* have to go on a diet again. Explain to them that this *is it*. If they just help you through this one last time, they'll never have to pull you through another diet again. Because you'll never put weight back on and thus have to lose it and drive them crazy again.

But don't put all the blame for your past failures on your family. You might as well admit to yourself that there were times that you used your family to keep you from dieting. Sometimes it was with excuses like "I had better go off this diet becase the starvation is making me so irritable I'm lashing out at the kids." But more often, it

267

was because you convinced yourself that you were unselfishly helping your family when you prepared snacks for your children or your spouse—a good portion of which you doubtlessly ate yourself.

Support can come from various directions, and it's up to you to enlist it. The society of other people is most crucial. We know that bingeing is a solitary activity while Staying Thin demands center stage. So as that Inner You begins emerging, make new friends. Other people can provide the positive reinforcement you need to keep your motivation high. Besides which, they provide a distraction. And if you can meet others in the same boat and keep company with, it's a valuable experience. (A little healthy competition never hurt anyone.) If you know someone who's also lost weight and kept it off, don't be afraid to share your experiences.

If you're out shopping alone, you might succumb to the temptation of grabbing a pizza, but if you're with a friend who's also resisting, you most likely won't. If your better half is in the kitchen with you while you're preparing dinner, prove to her or him that you can mix, stir, simmer, and fry without reaching in to nibble a bit. Don't be afraid then to boast. Brag. Show off. Be proud. But not too much or there will be no one around to do it for the next time.

The ones who won't share your joy (at least for the first five times you go off about your new weight situation) are saboteurs—those who have something to fear from your weight loss, or think they do. Don't fret about it—or them. Human relations are tough any way you look at it. They may be a little tougher when you're dieting. But you can handle it.

Stay cool—and Stay Thin.

16
Three Tools
for
Staying Thin

For some people, simply making their lives richer and fuller, rearranging their eating habits and homes, and learning how to handle former pitfalls will be enough to make them Stay Thin. They'll feel satisfied, they'll feel better about themselves, and they'll just naturally forget about their food compulsions. Those are the lucky ones; and they're not exactly typical.

Most compulsive eaters, however, need more thought and work to root the problem out and make sure the solution sticks. A good way to begin is to take another long hard look at yourself.

I don't mean this as a figure of speech. I mean you have to gauge accurately, with mirrors, scales, and food diaries, how you really look, how much you weigh, what you actually eat, how much you actually eat, and when and why you eat it.

If you don't give yourself this kind of feedback about your looks and your habits, it's all too easy to deceive yourself. "Oh I'm only a little overweight," or "I eat so little, I don't know where the pounds are coming from." Are you ready to face the truth?

If you are, your first tool is your mirror. Chances are strong that if you have a weight problem, there are very few mirrors around your house. Furthermore, there are probably no full-length mirrors there at all, or if there is one, it's stuck in a place where you can only see half of yourself, and then only if you're standing at some difficult angle. And no doubt, it's in a room you rarely enter.

Thin people constantly check themselves in mirrors, admiring the image. It isn't just narcissism; their self-love serves a positive purpose: putting themselves in condition for the rest of the world to love them. Physically, they check to see that everything's in place: buttoned, combed, and neat. Psychologically, they go over themselves for flaws, for aspects of their character that can stand improvement. They want to please others and know that the way to achieve that is by making sure they please themselves first.

But overweight people have thrown in the sponge. Having given up on pleasing others, they don't bother to please themselves either. Once this line is drawn, they can wallow in self-loathing and self-abnegation. They stop caring for themselves.

271

They stop looking in real mirrors and create a fantasy of what they look like. In their mental mirrors, they see only an image that never changes, no matter what form the external self takes. In other words, they look past their fat and see the image of a nice, thin, fascinating person. If their face is thin, they don't look below it; if their face is fat, they focus on their lovely eyes.

This didn't happen to them—or you—overnight. As your weight increased, you began to ignore real mirrors, because they showed you someone you didn't want to see, someone you couldn't like any more. So you turned instead to the mirror in your mind, where you could see only the self you imagined.

Now is the time to put the mirrors up once again. Not just small ones, but big decorative mirrors where you can't miss seeing yourself—on the bathroom door, in the front hall, over the dining room table. There's nothing wrong with looking at yourself in the mirror. Seeing the real, thinner you will be one of the strongest motivations to keep you Staying Thin.

You might even do what Tom B. did after he lost 175 pounds (yes, he really did). He not only put in a full-length mirror in the bedroom, and one behind the bathroom door, but decorated the wall next to the refrigerator with mirrors to keep him from slipping from grace when he was alone in the kitchen.

Putting the mirrors back is just a small step. Now, look at them. Strip completely and gaze at yourself in a real looking glass. Look not at the person you'd like to see but at the person who's really there. What do you see? *Honestly?* Sagging thighs? Drooping buttocks? A belly that rolls over your waist?

Now, put on your undergarments. Even clothed, do you see the telltale signs of overweight? Puffed-out cheeks? Wrinkled, overly fleshy skin on your neck that reminds you of a turkey? More than one chin?

You can't carry a full-length mirror around with you, so imprint this image in your brain, strongly enough so that you can't forget how you really look now. This is how others see you. Believe me, they're not looking past that fat face for those lovely eyes.

You don't want them to see this real you. Which is one reason why you're planning to take the road to permanent slimness. Others don't like that real you either. And now that you've recognized that this stranger is yourself, you don't really like that person either.

Would you rather be a sight or a sight for sore eyes?

Your second tool is your scale. A scale is to a dieter what a thermometer is to a doctor. It can tell you how high the fever has gone. It can cheer you as it goes lower. And without it, you have an easy time convincing yourself that your pants don't fit because they shrank in the wash.

Keep a small notebook and a pencil next to the scale. Weigh yourself once a day, and write down your weight. It's foolish to push the panic button when subtle increases are registered (and on the other hand to celebrate with a candlelit cupcake when you've dropped a half a pound). Sometimes lost fat is temporarily replaced with water in the tissues, a condition that will correct itself if you continue to watch your weight. But if a slight weight gain lasts more than a few days, or worse still, seems to be increasing, it's time to return to a full-fledged diet.

And finally, your third and most important tool for losing weight is your food diary. Writing things down, whether triumphs or disasters, good news or bad, helps pinpoint your Achilles' heel as well as your progress, and helps you get a better perspective—and sometimes even a sense of relief. A food diary is a tried-and-true method of behavior-modification weight-loss programs. Indeed, many people find it to be one of the most important steps to take.

Most compulsives are so used to automatically shoveling the food in that they don't really know what they're doing. Or how much they're taking in. The food diary, when properly kept, provides an accurate, bite-by-bite record of all the food that passes through your lips. If you keep it faithfully, there's no way to pretend, or truly believe, that you didn't have that extra serving of potatoes. Not to mention dessert. It's all there, in black and white.

Having to record what you're eating also serves as a reminder—as well as a restrainer. "I was ashamed," says Iris B., "when I realized how much food I was putting away. I didn't want to see 'four Oreos and three Cokes' in my food diary for an afternoon entry. So I cut them out, had broth instead, and felt virtuous."

Get yourself a notebook from the five and ten. After you eat anything, make the following notations in the book:

1. Time you ate.
2. What you ate.
3. How much you ate.
4. How hungry you were (on a scale of 1 to 5).
5. Where you ate it.
6. With whom you ate.
7. Under what circumstances you ate (e.g., how you were feeling at the time, did someting happen right before to upset you, etc.).

Then once a week, carefully go over this list. Study it. See if you can find a pattern emerging. If so, do something about it—fast—before it gets out of hand.

When you fill in the chart, don't guess or approximate. This is critical. Be exact about the time and place where you ate. Were you at home? Were you alone or did you have company? Were you just eating or were you doing something else at the same time—reading, watching TV, or talking on the phone?

Here are some of the things you should look for on this list:

TIME

Would your eating habits improve if you were to change the time of a main meal? Is there some particular time of the day when you're most likely to go off your diet? For example, Alice F. saw that her worst time was right after her husband left for work and her children went off to school. On the other hand, John L. found that his most likely hour to slip was right after the workday was over, when he left the office and its pressures.

Once each person realized that these were rough times for them, they did something to change their patterns: Alice got a part-time job in the mornings, and John changed his route to the train station after work so he would no longer pass the candy store. It took him a little longer to get home, it's true, but he avoided temptation when his resistance was as its lowest ebb.

WHAT AND HOW MUCH YOU ATE

List exactly what you had to eat, and how much of it. Most people are so locked into the idea that they only eat three "meals" a day, they don't even remember to list all their in-between snacks. In fact, they're hardly aware of eating them. Be aware. That's what Staying Thin is all about. List every lousy potato chip that you grab out of someone else's snack as you pass his desk in the office, every "little bite" someone offers you (and you take), every mint you pick up at the check-out counter. Be scrupulously honest.

Irene H., for example, knew that she was fallng off her diet many afternoons, but she felt that it wasn't that serious a problem since she would just nibble on a few items and never finish anything. As a result, she couldn't figure out why she was putting on so much weight. But when she honestly recorded how much she was eating, she was astounded: things like three quarters of a bag of potato chips *plus* a half a bag of pretzels in a single afternoon. She had been deluding herself that because she never finished a bag of anything, she was merely sampling and not glutting out.

If you keep your diary regularly, can't seem to Stay Thin, and don't understand what's wrong with any of these food entries, it may help to have a friend look it over for you. He or she may notice something you overlooked. "I had completely forgotten," says Dave L., "that orange juice has calories. I just thought of it as a good healthy drink and a natural source of Vitamin C. So I drank it whenever I was thirsty." David's friend Phil pointed out to him that all the Vitamin C he needed was available in a tablet, with none of the calories. And David also switched to tea.

Juice, in fact, has been unmasked as a culprit in many dieters' diaries. Fresh fruit is a far better choice, providing filling pulp and the chance to get in some chewing or all-important oral gratification. But with juice, a few quick swallows and it's all gone—except from your waistline.

WHERE YOU ATE
This is likely to pinpoint two problem areas: outside eating and in-home snacking. If you note that you're frequently cheating at a particular fast-food place, you may be able to change your route to avoid it. Or simply declare it out of bounds and refuse to stop there at all.

Another thing the details of where you ate may reveal is that you're frequently eating away from the dining room. In front of the TV for instance. Or in the garden while you're cutting the lawn. Or in bed.

UNDER WHAT CIRCUMSTANCES

Part of this is physical, like with whom you ate, what you were doing at the time, whether it was a regularly scheduled meal, etc. But it's the psychological part that is the most crucial, because that helps you understand under what conditions you are most likely to go overboard. This, as we discussed earlier, will help you be prepared for snacks and binges and come up with alternate behavior patterns.

The reason you're overeating may not be immediately clear to you after only one week, since the roots of overeating are complicated. Don't be surprised if it takes longer for your particular pattern to emerge from the record.

Dorothy G., for instance, found that she frequently did extra-curricular nibbling right before her daughter Janet came home from school at three, and after ten when her daughter went to bed. In one case, she recorded that she "didn't feel right about Janet." On another occasion, in which she had an all-out binge at 2 P.M. she wrote that she felt "harried from all the demands Janet made on me." She also noted frequent entries of "low," "blue," "guilty," "slightly anxious," and so on.

After looking through several notations like this, and rereading the chapter "How Your Compulsive Eating Began," she began to get the picture: it was anxiety about her daughter—of whom she had a great deal of unconscious jealousy—that was pinching her tail. Once she recognized this, she was able to prepare a different and a better response to this family problem. And she got so hooked on diary keeping that she began to keep a real nonfood diary to ventilate her other problems, such as her ambivalence about her daughter. (Both helped her weight problem.)

HOW HUNGRY WERE YOU

After two weeks, Rick J. was surprised to find far more entries marked "1" or "not hungry at all" than anything else. So he began to add more to his list of what he was feeling. It turned out that boredom was the usual culprit. "Now, when I feel like a snack, I try to listen to my stomach," he says. "I say 'Hey stomach, was that you calling me?' If it wasn't, I ignore the signal and try to find something besides eating to counteract the boredom." (A good place for him to start would be chapter 7.) Rich also started making his lunch hours later, so that he was hungrier, which also took care of at least one afternoon snack.

"Listening to your stomach" is really hard for compulsive overeaters because they're actually never hungry. "Now wait a minute," you may be saying to yourself. "I'm hungry all the time," But once you get the food diary habit, you may see that that's not true at all. Many compulsive overeaters never give themselves the chance to be really hungry because they've always got their mouths and stomachs full.

At the end of the week, study your charts carefully. Analyze the problems in your eating behavior. Is there a particular time of the day when you're vulnerable? A particular place? Does a particular person lead you down the wrong path? Does a TV show, or a phone call from your mother-in-law, or some other specific situation trigger a binge, or even the desire for a binge? Be your own detective; your own stern parent.

When you've finished your analysis, write down your findings, just the way a doctor might write up a case history of a patient. Some people really get into this. Hal H. says, "Afterwards, I take a separate color magic marker for each category and chart it week by week. Then I can really see the progress I'm making."

All three tools—your mirror, your scales, and your food diary—will give you the feedback you need about your individual eating snags and problems. But they'll do more than just that. The food diary will give you discipline—and discipline is what a compulsive overeater lacks.

Furthermore, they'll sharpen your desire to lose weight. They'll help you find out where you've been going wrong. They'll point out the right way to go. And as you lose weight, they'll offer tangible proof that you're doing it. Every time you look in that mirror, or step on that scale, or look into that diary, you'll feel better about your newly emerging permanently thin self.

17
ESTABLISHING REWARDS

Still another major way to ensure that you'll travel the straight and narrow path—the Stay Thin Road—is to develop a system of rewarding yourself.

Over the years, a growing body of psychological studies has highlighted the value of giving oneself rewards for changing behavior patterns. Of course, we use rewards in many ways throughout our lives. We all have our little private arrangements. For instance, we might tell ourselves that if we work hard all week, we'll give ourselves a special treat on the weekend—like going out to dinner and the theater.

Unfortunately, for many of us, eating gets tangled up in our rewards system, and this usually dates back to childhood. Mothers tell their children that if they behave well, they'll be rewarded with candy, or a trip to the ice cream store. A student will promise himself a pizza when he finishes his homework. A housewife will set aside a shopping day—and lunch—as a reward for those long, long days of motherhood. So, that's something to beware of.

What you must do is develop a whole system of nonfood rewards. In this way, you develop self-reliance on your efforts, gain control over your eating behavior, and get some enjoyment and pleasure in the bargain. You need support in your battle against excess eating. It can come from within you. The trade-off will not only help you feel and look better, it will make you think more highly of yourself.

Let's use an example. Jill T. is a magazine reporter who has an eating problem. Every afternoon, she compulsively eats candy and junk food, facing down her deadline. "I had quit smoking and found that as the pressure mounted to get the story in, I would start reaching for something to put in my mouth." The conflict, however was making her very unhappy and adding inches to her waistline. Chewing gum was a good stopgap. But, more importantly, she developed a system of rewards to help circumvent the eating mania. She calculated that she consumed about $2.00 worth of food while at the typewriter. She now decided that she'd take that money and put it to another, better use. It would pay for the ballet lessons that she had always wanted to take. She had calculated that the weekly tab for her junk-food habit would bankroll two lessons a week. Today, she is happy that she made the decision: she enjoys the ballet, she's losing weight, but best of all she has a feeling of being in control, of having made a choice and stuck to it.

Frances M. is another example. She has an enormous record collection but she always seems to want more, and it's hard to fit them into her budget. So, she has devised a rather complicated, mathematical system for buying new records. She puts aside one dollar for every half-pound she loses; and an extra two dollars at the end of every week when her weight stays stable. If she gains a pound, she forfeits the two dollars. I think she gets more pleasure out of her calculations than she does from listening to the records, but Frances swears by her system. "It makes me feel that I'm in business with myself. I strike bargains, I win, I lose—and I get a reward. It makes me feel good," she says happily.

What we call "self-control' is very related to the whole reward issue. It's not unusual for a person who is intelligent and rational to engage in behavior that endangers his health and generates frustration and misery for him. Like overeating. Others (and perhaps he or she as well) tend to attribute this behavior to the lack of willpower in his or her psychological make-up. Thus, the overweight person who is unable to shed excess weight is condemned as one who cannot muster enough willpower or self-control to stop eating.

The existence or nonexistence of something called "willpower" or "self-control," however, cannot be explained so easily. According to traditional beliefs, all one allegedly has to do to resist a temptation is to summon one's inner strength, an independent force that has its own existence. Just call upon your willpower and lo and behold, it bounces into action, transcends all frustrations, and resists temptation for the party.

To simplify things a bit, let's take a hypothetical example of someone without "willpower," and what you will see is that what he or she's really lacking is an ability to visualize or handle rewards.

Mrs. Jones would love to lose forty pounds during the next six months. She is highly motivated to lose this weight. She talks enthusiastically about her forthcoming diet to her husband and her friends. She thinks, even dreams, of the rewards of losing those terrible unwanted pounds, of being slim once more, praised by her husband, friends, and children, feeling attractive, and enjoying a better sex life. In short, she's about as psyched up to lose those forty pounds as anybody can be.

She decides on what diet she will use and immerses herself in this new program like an athlete training for the Olympics. However, unlike the athlete, after a few days of rigorous self-denial, Mrs. Jones decides that she can no longer continue. Sadly, she laments that "I just don't have the willpower for it any more."

Now that's the way she explains her failure. But if you delve deeper into why she quit her diet, another picture emerges. She first fell off the food wagon when she was shopping with a friend and they decided to have lunch in the department store restaurant. At the next table, Mrs. Jones saw the waitress bring a sundae to a middle-aged woman just like herself. It was Mrs. Jones' favorite type of sundae too—hot fudge.

Here are the types of thoughts Mrs. Jones began to have. "She's doing it. Why shouldn't I have one, too? That woman can eat all she wants. I can't. Why not? It's not fair. In other ways she seems to be like me. But I'm the one who has to suffer. I'll always have to suffer because of this damned weight problem. Already, I've been suffering again for six days. And what have I gotten in return? I lost one lousy pound. Ninety-five percent of my waking thoughts in the last six days have been about food and I dreamt about it too. But all I got for my diet was a lot of frustration and tension. What's the use of even trying? It just isn't fair."

Now at this point she had a conflict. She wanted the sundae—but she also wanted to lose forty pounds. So what made her choose the sundae?

"My mouth started watering when I looked at it," she might have said, "I found myself salivating at the sight of it. I tasted it long before I even took the first spoonful."

Now, think for a moment of what was really taking place. Mrs. Jones looked at a chocolate sundae. Behold. It looked luscious. Her mouth watered. She wanted to get her teeth into it. To anticipate tasting the ice cream sundae was immediately rewarding. The desirable consequences of eating the sundae could be experienced right at that moment, whereas the consequences of losing forty pounds could only be experienced in the future. Everyone knows that when faced by an immediate reward situation and a future reward possibility, it's a rare person who defers the immediate reward. And it is often this conflict between a short-term reward and a long-term one which is what traditionalists call "willpower" or "self-control"—simply the ability to postpone the immediate reward for the later one.

To eat something **now** produces immediately satisfying consequences. To think of future satisfactions brings pleasure too, albeit to a much lesser degree. In addition, denying yourself the immediate reward may also produce actually negative consequences such as headaches, tiredness, sullenness, not to mention hunger.

Is it any wonder that so many people choose to eat **now** and to reward themselves **now**, to forestall unpleasant consequences **now**?

This present-future conflict, as you can see, is quite different from what is ordinarily believed to be willpower or self-restraint. It does not, by any stretch of the imagination, involve an independent force within the individual that is arbitrarily called upon to function. It is merely a matter of people doing what they do many times every day of their lives—deciding between rewards now or later.

If you give it some thought, you'll soon realize that almost all of our goals are rewarded not now, but in the future. People go to work, not because they'll be paid at the end of each hour, but perhaps two weeks later. A man regularly takes out a young woman whom he hopes he might marry one day, even though it won't happen for months, maybe years. A mother gets up early each morning and drives her children to school, although it may be years before she sees the concrete results of any learning.

If you stopped and thought of how often we defer present leasure for future gain, it might be far simpler for you to do so in food-related situations as Miss Jones should have done. All she had to say to herself was "I choose long-terms goals in most other situations. I can do it here too." After all, she was not weak and lacking in "willpower" in other life situations, so why should she have trouble with this?

It helps to think also about something that could make it easier for you to maintain your weight goal: giving yourself more rewards NOW for turning down food. Don't let the thin you of the future be the sole reward. In many cases, for most people, it is not enough.

You, and others, devise such reward-exchanges every day. For instance, a worker decides that he's been laboring hard, and that after he gets his raise, he's going to take two weeks off and have a real vacation. Or a student decides that after he finishes writing that tough paper, he'll vedge out on TV for an hour.

In thousands of instances like the above, a contingency relationship is set up between some desirable or required activity and a reward whose realization depends upon the performance of the activity. When you perform X, you are allowed to do Y. Typical examples:

X	Y
Work at your job.	Receive pay check.
Save money.	Buy a stereo.
Clean the house.	Go shopping.
Exercise daily.	Maintain weight.

It is important for you to establish a contingency relationship between your eating behavior and self-reward. This process leads to greater self-control and self-management, and less dependence on others. By creating contingencies between your eating behavior and the rewards, you can exercise enormous control over your food intake.

What kinds of rewards should you use? Anything which is pleasant for you. As long as it's not food. You can even use reward activities which you customarily take for granted, but get a lot of pleasure out of, such as telephoning a friend, watching a favorite program on TV, going to a movie, buying something new.

Later, weeks from now, or months from now, you will find that you're able to substitute a symbolic reward for an actual, material one. That is, you will be able to feel so good about yourself that that will be reward enough. At this time, you need more, however. And don't rush it. Each person has different needs and yours may be greater than others'.

Every week that Diana stays at her ideal weight of 112, she puts aside $3.00 which will be used to purchase a new dress.

When Anne eats her dinner slowly, chewing and tasting every morsel instead of gulping it down like she used to, she rewards herself with a second cup of coffee.

Every day that Joan doesn't snack between meals entitles her to watch one more hour of TV.

When Sam eats raw vegetables and unbuttered popcorn instead of fattening snacks, he treats himself to a bucket of golf balls at the driving range that evening.

Some people, of course, have eccentric tastes. Arlene B. is a cotton lover. She can't stand to wear anything made from fake fabrics, like polyester, and she can't stand to sleep on wash-and-wear sheets. So, when she's particularly pleased with herself, she treats herself to a new set of all-cotton sheets. They're expensive, but they feel wonderful to her. To another person, new sheets might seem like a mundane sort of treat, but to Arlene, they spell luxury and a sense of well-being.

And remember to be well aware, always, of the difference between the immediate and the long-term reward. Faced by a reward now versus a reward later, most people would succumb to the immediate one. Waiting till later is what "will-power" is all about.

A system of rewards or substitute gratifications will help keep temptation at arm's length. It can focus your mind away from the scene of your potential downfall. Setting up a long-range goal can also provide you with a handy vision of what you are striving for as you ride along the bumpy road to self-control—and to Staying Thin.

18
Staying Thin

Staying Thin and creating a new body is a process—a long one, a rewarding one and one into which you just have to put a great deal of effort. You're thin now. But Staying Thin, that is something else again.

In the early part of this book, it was explained how feeling bad can put weight on you. Ironically, so can feeling good. Many people, when they reach their desired weight, become so elated that they forget they still have (and always will have) a weight problem. They soon slip back into their old ways—hurrying through meals, snaking while watching TV, allowing themselves the luxury of a late-night pig-out whenever the mood strikes. Then one day, they're fat again.

It isn't enough to make changes for a week or two; you have to commit yourself for a lifetime. On the plus side, though, I promise you it will get easier. After a while, some of the changes in your eating patterns will become second nature to you. In time, you'll eat the Stay Thin way without even thinking about it. You'll be in control—at the controls—and you'll be able to switch yourself onto automatic pilot. You won't have to worry about food all the time. But it won't happen overnight. It may take months, even years, before your good eating habits become as automatic to you as your wrong ones were.

Meanwhile, guard against backsliding. Weigh yourself at least once a week. If you don't take a hard look at that scale regularly, it becomes easy to close your eyes to the pounds when they start creeping up on you again. Look back over the lists you've made in the course of reading this book, and keep an ongoing analysis of your food diary.

Don't ever start thinking wistfully back to the days when you could eat whatever you wanted to. Look at what happened to you as a result. And stop referring to your old condition as "solid" or "big boned." You were fat. Say it to yourself again and again. It's not a pleasant thought— which is why if you admit its veracity, you're less likely to return to that odious condition.

In its place, try being thin. If you don't like it, you have the option of changing. You already know how easy it would be to get fat again. As one man, who has kept his 120-pound weight loss for eight months now, says, "I know I'm always just a mouthful away from having to start all over again."

To make sure this doesn't happen to you, at least once every few months, for the next couple of years, go to a department store, visit the beach or cruisewear section, and look at yourself in a three-way mirror, under those awful lights—in a bathing suit. Often our eyes can show us what a scale can't, and when we're completely dressed with only small mirrors around, we don't even see the fat starting in the first place. But those three-way mirrors do.

And don't forget exercise. Remember, that doesn't have to mean sweating and straining. It doesn't have to involve weekly exercise classes, daily jogging, or frequent laps in the swimming pool, if you're not quite up to it yet. Just break a few of your lazier habits by doing at least some of the following:

*If you live or work on a low floor, walk up and down the stairs instead of taking the elevator.
*Stop looking for the closest parking space—walk a bit of a distance to your car.
*Instead of ordering lunch, go out and buy it.
*Get off buses one stop before your destination.

Now, these may not seem like very big deals, and they're not, but they can add up. Two or three extra city blocks a day of walking can add up to about fifty miles a year. So sit down and think of everything you do on a weekday, and on a weekend day. Then think about how you could sneak a little more exercise into some of those activities.

And while you're at it, sneak in some really pleasurable ones as well. Rediscover sex. Maybe you avoided lovemaking because you felt like—maybe looked like—Henry VIII or Kate Smith.

Now you're slim. And it's time to get a sitter for the weekend while you go off to check into a motel for a re-creation of your honeymoon.

Rediscover the joy of physical freedom and activity. Before you became slim, you weren't muscle-bound, you were blubber-bound. You couldn't play Ping-Pong without panting after a few rounds. You couldn't even aspire to touch football. Or jog without embarrassment. But now, there's no extra poundage to hold you back. So take off; choose your sport and tear into it.

Use the drives and energies that caused you to overeat for other purposes. Don't hire someone to finish the basement. Think of the pleasure—and pride—you'll feel when you do it yourself. The same thing goes for painting the kitchen, making a child's rocker for an expected grandchild, or turning part of the cellar into a darkroom and developing your own pictures.

REMEMBER THE WHY

Self-esteem affects every aspect of your life, waking and even sleeping. (Studies of the sleep of those who have low self-esteem show that they are more likely to suffer from insomnia.) And what unites members of the obese fraternity is a low self-esteem, a feeling of inadequacy, both about their bodies and about their minds. Remember? Isn't it true that when you were fat, you weren't really happy with yourself? There wasn't a jolly inner person under all that flab, now was there?

Learning self-love is the start of the long road back. Learning to view yourself as worthwhile, as attractive, as whatever you want to be, is a giant step. For that old equation works both ways, if you tell a person often enough that he looks good—and, more importantly, if he starts to tell himself that he does—sooner or later he'll oblige you—and himself—by looking good. Self-fulfilling prophecies can work any way you like. But until then, every Kodak Instamatic is like a dagger, every mirror a criminal conviction, and the obese person goes through life like a soldier inching through a minefield.

Isn't it great to be liberated from all that? Well, soldier, let me give you this simple reminder: once you reach your final goal, it doesn't mean that you've won, that the fight is over. You've just won the battle. Now you have to fight the war.

One reason many people lose the war is because of the "if-I-ever-lose-weight" syndrome. Chances are that when you were overweight, you spent a lot of time convincing yourself that if you ever really lost weight, life would be a whole lot different. You'd have more friends. You'd have more dates. You'd go to more parties. You'd do better in work. You'd get a better job. And so on. Ad nauseum. Literally.

Well, now you are thin. And temporarily at least, things may even seem to be a little worse. You may have lost a few friends while you were losing those pounds. Maybe they became jealous and ditched you. Or your dropped them when you realized they were using you, because when you were fat, and had low self-esteem, you allowed those things to happen.

Furthermore, your business may have dropped off a little in the past few months because you placed dieting above everything else. Or you were crabby and difficult to be with and lost a few points as a result.

So the miracles you were expecting did not occur the moment you hit your goal weight. But the first thing you are going to have to do now is to realize that your former goals were probably wildly unrealistic in the first place. And they therefore need to be scaled down.

For example, women, just because you lost forty pounds this year doesn't mean that man who looks like Robert Redford you've had a crush on all year is now going to ask you out.

And men, no matter how much weight you lost this year, and how good a baseball player you were when you were young (before you put on all that weight), you're not going to be pitching for the Yankees this year. Or anything like it.

And don't go stuffing your face in disappointment. What you expected to occur happens to very few people—thin or fat. And the reason those things didn't come about for you had nothing to do with your weight.

So your next step—rather than giving up altogether—is to start setting more realistic goals. Think back to some of your more grandiose fantasies. Start scaling them down. So you secretly fantasized that you would be president of your company if only you were thin. Maybe you will be one day. But would you be satisfied now with a nice raise this year? That may not seem like much compared to what you had dreamed of. But isn't it probably more than what you would have gotten if you had stayed fat?

Or maybe you single women expected to go out every night once you became thin. But if you go out now once or twice a week (and with real people, not with the unrealistically fantastic dates you once envisioned were out there), aren't you still better off than you were before?

Most "swingers" don't become that way overnight anyway. It took them years of dating before they developed the social skills and contacts that brought them a lot of dates and made them at ease when they were out with members of the opposite sex. So don't expect to make an immediate splash when you dive into the social pool now.

In fact, lack of experience can even be a plus for you. Carole Y. found that rather than floundering on dates, it was helpful to honestly admit that she was new at the game. "When Carl came to pick me up that first night, I was petrified," she remembers. "I was twenty-six years old and had gone out exactly twice in my fat life—and both times I was under sixteen."

"Everything went wrong. I wasn't sure with women's lib whether I was supposed to open my own door, or wait for him to do it. So I waited for a couple of seconds, nothing happened, so I moved for the door. Simultaneously, so did he, I hit my nose, and got a nose bleed. And to top it off, I spilled the wine on the tablecloth reaching for the menu.

"It was such a disaster, that I decided to level

with him. I told him that I used to have a weight problem (I didn't think a first date was a good time to tell him that I used to weigh 200 pounds), and had become so self-conscious and shy that I never went out, and was still a social and sexual virgin. But then I told him I was glad I was trying my first date with him because I was really enjoying myself, and he was so comfortable to be around. Well, he just ate it up," she chuckled.

So, scale down your goals and be grateful for what you're getting. Appreciate the positive—if small—changes that are already occurring in your life. More—and better—things will continue to happen. But if you expect too much, you'll end up running back to the comfort and warmth of a seven-layer cake or whatever. And then these changes in your life will not occur at all.

Yes, you've made changes. But you're going to have to stick with them for the rest of your life. The moment you decide that it's all right to revert to the past—even for just one meal—because you're slim and it doesn't really matter any more, disaster looms.

No, you can't get rid of the temptations, because they will always be there. You will have to go through your whole life resisting banana splits, but that's no more difficult than the recovered alcoholic going through his or her whole life watching other people hoist martinis and guzzle cold beer. After a while, drinking is simply not as attractive as sobriety is, and there are also some pretty positive rewarding reasons for Staying Thin: attractive clothes, good health, admiration, etc. Just think of the day when they will no longer be inaccessible jewels locked inside a glass case, reminders of your inadequacy.

So make no mistake about it. Temptation will never go away. There's not an escalator in the world without a stairway somewhere nearby, and whenever you come to one of those you'll have to choose. Will you opt for the stairs? Or will you tell yourself it doesn't matter, you can ride up with a machine doing the work your legs should be doing? Take-the-easy-way choices will confront you forever, so you'll have to learn to spot yourself in the act of self-betrayal. You can never let down your guard.

You'll hit snags along the way; moods are a difficulty. They vary. Temptation is strong one day, weak the next. Resentment against the whole damned subject of weight loss is a familiar problem; people get sick and tired of being careful.

But one of the greatest kinds of satisfaction is that which comes from directing yourself up the path of virtue rather than down the primrose path of dalliance: to go out with a friend and just have black coffee while he or she devours a banana split can give rise to some very positive, very virtuous feelings.

Don't kid yourself that swearing off your past way of life isn't going to be traumatic. For being overweight is gratifying, simple, passive. And Staying Thin is tough.

No one can help you if you don't care. That is the bottom line. Just remember: Your appearance does matter. It affects every aspect of your life:

physical emotional, romantic, professional, and social. If it's a real pleasure being mayor in a city of one, if you find it easy to ignore the siren call of the outside world, O.K. But resign yourself now to staying fat forever. No program you go on, no book you read, no system you adopt will magically do it for you.

TAKE GOOD CARE OF ALL OF YOURSELF

When you don't dress right, or wear the proper clothes or hair style, you're advertising that you don't feel right about yourself. That there's something that keeps you from putting your best foot forward. Or that you don't have a best foot to put forward.

An important first step in Staying Thin is to get a new wardrobe to match your new body. Many people who lose weight continue to wear their old clothes, almost as a source of pride. Seeing how big their pants are reminds them constantly of how little their body is. But ill-fitting clothes detract from your new good looks. It looks bad to others when you turn your back and the seat of your pants is baggy. Or when people look at your neck and see something scraggly emerging from your collar.

Furthermore, new, attractive clothes that fit keep you slim. They make you look better, so you're more likely to get compliments, and to protect your investment by making sure you don't grow out of them.

Along with the new clothes, get a new haircut and styling. Chances are your face is slimmer now; you may be able to wear a style you couldn't get away with before. Women might do well to go to a department store and get a free makeup job. Or, if you're a man—or the type of woman who never wears makeup—buy yourself a new hat.

In addition, spend some money now on something that will last—and ultimately help you. Throw your old clothes away, and buy a new coat, a suit, an evening dress, something you really don't want to grow out of.

If you're the sort of person—and there are many of these—who simply don't care about clothes, and who go around in a kind of uniform, which they replenish only when it wears out and falls apart, beautify whatever it is that you *do* care about. Reupholster a chair, buy a new lithograph for your office wall, invest in some exotic houseplants. But do try to make your rewards personal.

A new garage door, for instance, while undeniably useful and necessary, is not the way to reward yourself for successfully exercising often ornery willpower. Now is the time to indulge yourself—clothes, beauty aids, flowers—something that will make you, or your surroundings, more pleasant to the eye. Car repairs, kitchen appliances, a new exterminator for the nest of wasps under the eaves—these are not rewards for Staying Thin.

Take the long view too. Chances are that you're more than just looking good, you're feeling a whole lot better. And people are saying good things to you. Maybe people of the opposite sex are looking at you with renewed interest.

But these external supports probably won't last. People forget. If your weight stays the same, they'll quit commenting on it, and take it for granted. Even the high you're feeling now as a result of your incredible accomplishment is likely to wear off.

So plan something a couple of months from now that's likely to give you a lift. It can be a vacation—if you think you can handle it without overeating. Maybe that's the time to get the new stereo you wanted. Or you might decide that two or three months from now would be a good time to look up that old beau.

These long term plans will help you get over a period when you might possibly slip, a plateau, for example.

Again—and this is the last time you'll hear this—awareness of your problems, your personality structure, your way of handling stress, is half the battle. And once you're aware you can start dealing, intelligently, with the lifelong project of Staying Thin. Just look at what you've done already!

So promise yourself, and keep to it, that you're going to Stay Thin forever.

19
Thirty Days That Lead
to a Lifetime
of Staying Thin

By now, you should be at your goal weight, looking slim, feeling great, and anxious to stay that way. Forever. But what are you going to do to ensure that The New You lasts for a lifetime? How are you going to make certain that this time really is IT and you don't slip back?

Patients in our Stay Thin Programs have found that when they've reached their goal weight, and learned to live and eat the Stay Thin way, they can permanently "seal in" the changes by adhering faithfully to the following maintenance program for at least a month. After that, hopefully you'll follow it forever, but first things first.

STEP ONE: MAINTENANCE
The first thing I want to do is recapitulate a few

specific items I have already discussed in the book. Repetition may be tedious, but it's also necessary that the following tasks are strictly performed if you really want to Stay Thin. Make sure you do each and every one for the next thirty days faithfully so that they become a lifelong habit.

MIRROR: Every day for the rest of your life, you should take out a few seconds in the morning to look at yourself in a full-length mirror—with no clothes on. (Every once in a while, remember to go to the cruisewear section of a department store, try on a bikini, and look at yourself in a three-way mirror.)

FOOD DIARY: You learned on pages 273-280 how to keep a food diary. Now, each evening, look over this diary and critically evaluate how you fared. Start by comparing it to the food plan you are using, either yours or the one I suggested earlier. How close is your diet to your food plan? Where have you gone wrong? How could you improve? Are you eating when you're not really hungry? Sneaking in a few snacks that you could (and should) live without? Are you eating because you're anxious or talking on the phone? After you've gone over your food diary, write down the patterns, problems, etc. After a few days, you'll see patterns that should be worked on this month if you want to Stay Thin for the rest of your life.

ACTIVITIES PLANNED: Like planning your food in advance, planning your activities in the beginning can help keep you out of trouble. A great deal of mindless, needless snacking and even bingeing occurs when you have nothing else to do.

So make sure you plan each day to do something in the evenings, not to mention those few empty hours when you get home from work, and especially during the weekends. These are times when even the most dedicated dieters have downfalls.

SPORTS: During your thirty-day maintenance program, you should figure out what sports interest you and would be feasible for you to do. Plan a weekly schedule now that includes time for that sport at least twice a week—and don't wait any longer to make your first appointment.

REFRIGERATOR: By the end of each day, all the tempting foods in your refrigerator should have been wrapped and marked, low-calorie snacks should have been placed up front, no leftovers should have been left over, and, if you're a midnight binger, the lightbulb should have been removed from the refrigerator. Get into the lifetime habit of doing these things by working hard at it this month.

MEASURING YOUR WEIGHT: Weigh yourself before breakfast and then register the weight on a daily chart. If it's up for a day or two, don't panic. But if it stays up, ask yourself if you've been regularly exercising, planning your food intake in advance, planning your free-time activities, keeping your food diary conscientiously, participating in some sport regularly, etc.

STEP TWO: COPING WITH THE EXTERNAL ENVIRONMENT
Take this simple test and see whether you're still having trouble with the external environment. Ask

yourself if the following things are true for you and even if something is only true occasionally, consider it true.

I shop when I run out of food.

I don't prepare a shopping list.

When I shop, I buy food with the indefinite future in mind.

I go into the supermarket and/or food stores more than twice a week.

If I can't decide whether to buy an item, I'll examine the package.

While I'm standing at the check-out counter, I'll pick up some last minute items.

I like to look around the kitchen to see what I can find.

I like to grab leftovers from the refrigerator.

I nibble while I'm preparing food.

I nibble when I'm on the phone.

I eat in several places throughout the house.

I eat in more than one place in the house.

I have a phone and/or a TV in the kitchen.

There is one or more food place which I can't resist.

I snack while I'm watching TV.

I get up during commercials to see what's in the refrigerator.

I snack when I'm reading and/or studying.

When I'm in a restaurant, I forget about my diet.

I usually order the special dinner in restaurants.

When I'm on vacation I forget about my diet.

I have a tendency to overeat during the holidays.

There is at least one person who gets me to eat more than I had planned to.

When I invite people over, we invariably eat.

I have dinner or lunch even if I'm not hungry.

I eat at my desk during lunch.

I stop eating when my plate is clean.

There's food around the house I shouldn't eat.

Now, if you answered "true" for just one question, then you're still having trouble with the external environment and could easily fall off the food wagon if you don't handle that problem quickly. Now maybe that seems hard on you. But it isn't. Say it's true for you that you grab leftovers from the refrigerator. I can hear you saying, "Yeah, but I only do it occasionally." But all it takes is one time with half a leftover cake and your diet will be as finished as that cake. (Besides which, when you slip once, you have a tendency to then say whatthe-hell and do it again.) So you must make sure that no leftovers are ever left over in the refrigerator until Staying Thin becomes as ingrained as Being Fat once was.

Look over your results on the quiz and see what areas are still giving you problems. Then, go through the Table of Contents in this book and reread whichever chapters (8-14) would help you handle your specific problem with the external environment.

In addition, if any of the items below relate to an area in which you're having problems, do the Special Assignment some time this month.

SPECIAL ASSIGNMENT: KITCHEN (CLEANING) Clean out all your kitchen cupboards, along with your refrigerator so you get rid of all the wrong foods you've accumulated from your years of bad eating. Now make a list of the right foods and buy them.

SPECIAL ASSIGNMENT: KITCHEN (COVER REFRIGERATOR ITEMS) Buy wrapping paper and a pen and cover everything in the refrigerator and freezer that might tempt you. Mark what the items are so you don't have to open anything to find out what's in there.

SPECIAL ASSIGNMENT: SHOPPING PLAN Think about what you purchased the last time you went to the supermarket. Then, plan a sample list for the future. When doing this, picture the supermarket in your mind. Then, write down the items in the order in which you'll pass them so you can get out of the market as fast as possible. Decide the best time and day for you to shop each week, most important, when you won't be hungry. Figure out how you can cut down on trips to the supermarket (e.g., buy a memo pad and write down foods as you run out of them so you won't forget them the next time you go to the market).

SPECIAL ASSIGNMENT: TV SNACKING Write down which TV programs you usually watch each day and ascertain where you generally have problems with snacking. Decide what you are going to do in the future on difficult nights (e.g., save your dessert for a late night snack on a long TV evening, prepare raw vegetables early in the evening, exercise instead of eating during commercials, etc.).

SPECIAL ASSIGNMENT: SNACK DIARY Write a snack diary (two pages will do) of the times and situations that most often led you to snack in the past. What external situations (e.g., passing a particular store, having a jar of peanut butter in the house) have been most likely to set you off? Look for your general pattern.

Now what can you do to cut out unscheduled snacking? Can you change your route so you won't pass the stores that cause you problems? Can you start snacking only at certain times (say only on an even hour) and shaping your snacks (say half and half raw vegetables and snack)? Plan now how you're going to handle snacking in the future.

SPECIAL ASSIGNMENT: INTERPERSONAL RELATIONS Examine the motives of the people around you. How supportive of your weight goals is your family? Which of your friends are really helping you to Stay Thin? Could any of them be unconsciously sabotaging you?

Think about those people who, consciously or unconsciously, are making it difficult for you to Stay Thin. First, try to figure out their motives and where they're coming from. Then, decide the best way to handle them. Finally, practice aloud what you're going to say to someone who persistently foists food on you when you're trying to Stay Thin.

SPECIAL ASSIGNMENT: RESTAURANTS Analyze your dining-out patterns. Which restaurants give you trouble? Under what circumstances are you likely to slip? How are you going to handle restaurant dining in the future?

SPECIAL ASSIGNMENT: HOLIDAYS, PARTIES, AND SPECIAL EVENTS What holidays, special events, or parties are coming up that could make you slip? Christmas? A wedding? A cocktail party next Saturday night? Make a list of how you're going to handle each of these situations so you won't overeat.

SPECIAL ASSIGNMENT: VACATIONS What type of vacations have gotten you into trouble in the past? Where are you going to spend your vacation this year? How are you going to handle the eating problem? Make a list of specific options and solutions.

STEP THREE: COPING WITH THE PSYCHOLOGICAL ASPECTS OF STAYING THIN

Now, take this test and see if any of the following items are true for you:

When I am beset by problems, I turn to food.

I often suddenly get a craving for a particular food.

Sometimes I eat without even realizing I'm doing it.

Sometimes I start eating and I just can't stop.

Being overweight upsets someone close to me.

I go on midnight binges.

I sneak extra food in when no one sees me.

When I have nothing to do, I find myself eating.

I eat after I argue or fight with someone.

I eat when I'm angry at someone.

When I feel blue, I eat.

When I feel frustrated, I eat.

When I feel guilty, I eat.

When I feel anxious, I eat.

When I feel sorry for myself, I eat.

If you answered yes to any of these, then your eating is probably a response to your psyche rather than your stomach or environment. To help you understand why you're doing this, and what you can do about it, reread chapters 5, 6, and 7

In addition, do these Special Assignments sometime this month to help you cope with the psychological factors that are likely to prevent you from permanently Staying Thin.

SPECIAL ASIGNMENT: BINGEING: Write a binge diary (two pages will do) of when you binged in the past, when you first started, what times seem to be the worst for you, what emotions or problems generally triggered a binge, etc. Reread the diary and see if you can find a pattern.

SPECIAL ASSIGNMENT: BINGEING ALTERNATIVES Look over the binge diary and ask yourself what the bingeing accomplished—and how it harmed you—each time it happened in the past. Then, plan how you're going to change your thoughts and attitudes so that when the urge to binge (or for that matter, snack), strikes again you will be able to handle it this time.

SPECIAL ASSIGNMENT: SUBSTITUTES FOR BINGEING (AND SNACKING) I suggested in chapter 7 that you make a list of things that you like to do (read a particular magazine, call a favorite friend) to temporarily distract you from improper eating. If you didn't do this earlier, do it now. Set up a "distraction center" on the way to the kitchen.

SPECIAL ASSIGNMENT: FINDING MAJOR NEW INTERESTS

In order to make food less important in your world, you're going to have to find other interests to take its place. Decide this month what these are going to be and take steps to start getting involved in these new hobbies or interests. For example, send for an adult-education-class catalogue, sign up for music lessons, etc.

SPECIAL ASSIGNMENT: UNDERSTANDING SEXUAL RELATIONSHIPS Focus this month on how you used being overweight to avoid love and sexual relationships. Think back to all the important relationships you've had with members of the opposite sex, starting when you were young. What were you afraid of? Did being overweight help you avoid it? Did you pay too high a price for your fears? What did being overweight contribute to those relationships? How did it harm them? How do you plan to cope with fears of sexuality in the future?

STEP FOUR: MOTIVATION

You probably think that motivation to Stay Thin is not your problem any more. After all, you've read this whole book and God knows how many times you've tried to get thin in the past. But are you sufficiently motivated now? To Stay Thin, to work hard and constantly at it?

To find out, take this test and see if any of these are true for you.

Sometimes I wonder if it's worth all I'm going through to Stay Thin.

I was happier when I was fatter.

When I'm thin, I'm miserable.

I never worry about the physical dangers of being overweight.

I don't care that much how I look.

I don't care how I look at the beach in a bathing suit.

I don't care what other people say about me.

Being fat had more advantages than being thin.

If you answered yes to any of these, reread chapters 3, 4, and 16 and do these following Special Assignments:

SPECIAL ASSIGNMENT (SELF-APPRAISAL) Rather than waiting, go to a department store immediately and try on a bikini—or, if you're a male, a very brief pair of bathing trunks. Look at yourself carefully in the three-way mirror.

What areas still need work? What are you going to do about it? Start those additional exercises and a more stringent diet today.

SPECIAL ASSIGNMENT: CONCENTRATING ON THIN PEOPLE—TV Tonight, when you're watching TV, notice how all the attractive actors and actresses are thin. Note also how the comic and pathetic characters are often overweight.

SPECIAL ASSIGNMENT: CONCENTRATING ON THIN PEOPLE—MAGAZINES Look through some magazines today (you can thumb through them on the newsstand), and focus on the thinness of the models. Concentrate especially on their facial structure, and note how lack of fat enables their best features (cheekbones, eyes, etc.) to come out.

SPECIAL ASSIGNMENT: PEOPLE WATCHING Pay special attention today to the people you see walking along the street. Note how much better clothes look on slimmer people. Notice how much more self-confident the thinner people look. Stand by a hot dog stand and watch the overweight people wolfing down their meals. Ask yourself who looks better—and who are the ones whom others seem to admire and notice.

SPECIAL ASSIGNMENT: DANGERS OF OVERWEIGHT Go to the library and look up some of the consequences of the diseases that afflict overweight people. Learn about the problems and dangers of heart disease, diabetes, high blood pressure. etc. Go ahead—scare yourself. Then, think of how nice it will be not to have to worry about it any more.

SPECIAL ASSIGNMENT: FAT NOVEL Write a "fat novel" (two or three pages will do). Write down how you got overweight and how others helped you wreck your body. If your weight gains were cyclical, try to pinpoint the period of time and what seemed to set you off. Then, reread it and try to find a pattern. Finally, resolve to add a new chapter to your life by always Staying Thin.

SPECIAL ASSIGNMENT: ANALYZING YOUR BAD HABITS Write down ways in which you've allowed yourself to be a victim in life. Besides compulsive overeating, what other bad habits have turned you into a victim? What have you gained by them? What have you lost? Were they worth the price?

SPECIAL ASSIGNMENT: REWARDS Calculate how much money snacks, bingeing, and just plain overeating used to cost you on an average month. Choose a reward for yourself at the end of these thirty days, bought with the money you're going to save by proper eating. Then, choose something for yourself for one year from now.

SPECIAL ASSIGNMENT: STAYING THIN Write down all the advantages of Staying Thin. Think of the pride you will have in yourself. Think of how you will look. Concentrate on how you will feel. Keep this list someplace where you can look at it about once a month for the rest of your life.

Finally, there are going to be times in the next month—and indeed, throughout your life—when

315

you are simply going to want to eat something you shouldn't and the hell with everyone and everything and every diet.

The next time this happens—and every time afterwards—return to this page and use it as an index to the pages you should read before you do anything rash. The following are three ways to cope with the I-don't-give-a-damn-anymore crisis whenever it occurs.

EXERCISE: It often helps to do some exercises until the urge to eat passes. See chapter 3 for ten exercises that should keep your body instead of your mouth occupied.

ALTERNATIVE ACTIVITIES: On pages 133-140 you learned how to stop yourself from bingeing or snacking by doing other activities you enjoyed, and one of the Special Assignments during this thirty-day program was to make such a list if you hadn't done this already. Now reread those pages and turn to this list. Engage in one of these activities instead of eating.

TALKING TO YOURSELF: On pages 146-153 you learned what to say to yourself to stop yourself when you're about to grab food, e.g., how to maximize the problem, take it one day at a time, and change negative thinking. Reread these pages when you're about to overeat and apply these thoughts to yourself and your own food problem.

Although these are methods of coping with a crisis, it's really best to try to pinpoint problem areas long before they creep up on you. Will you soon be passing your favorite pizza stand on the way to your night course? Will tonight be a long evening of watching TV with lots of food commercials to tempt you? Are you likely to be a little depressed later tonight because this is the day each week that your elderly mother calls and complains that you don't see her frequently enough?

Of course not all problems, crises and temptations can be anticipated in advance. But when they can, don't wait until you're right in the pizza parlor to decide how you're going to handle them. Plan an alternate route now, or plan to have no money with you, or go to that area with a supportive friend. How are you going to handle the guilt or depression after your mother calls? With a binge? Or with a preplanned activity that will help pull you out of that weekly funk? Go over anticipated problems and plan in advance how you're going to cope with each one of them, and chances are, that later, the problem won't be very bad.

Make these changes in the next thirty days and a lifetime will be easy.

Good luck.

And Stay Thin.

FICTION FOR TODAY'S WOMAN

THE LAST CARESS (722, $2.50)
by Dianna Booher
When the news that their daughter might die transforms Erin's husband into a distant, isolated man, Erin learns that there is more than one way to lose someone you love—and few ways to win them back. . . .

TO SUFFER IN SILENCE (748, $2.75)
by Patricia Rae
The back ward of Harwell State Mental Hospital is a place no one will discuss. And Daniel, an invalid without the powers of speech or movement, is imprisoned there. Unable to convey his sanity, he is alone. Powerless, he is forced TO SUFFER IN SILENCE.

THE VOW (653, $2.50)
by Maria B. Fogelin
She was an exquisite bride-to-be, with the vigor and determination to make her dreams come true—until a devastating accident destroyed her future. Still, she found the courage to live, and searched for the courage to love.

CELEBRATE WHAT IS (764, $2.50)
by Doris Standridge
The true story of a mother's tragic inability to accept the invalid state of her once strong and athletic son—and of a young man's courageous battle for life!

SO LITTLE TIME (585, $2.50)
by Sharon Combes
Darcy's love and courage are put to the test when she learns that her fiance has only months to live. And the most important test of all, is the test of time. . . .

Available wherever paperbacks are sold, or order direct from the Publisher. Send cover price plus 50¢ per copy for mailing and handling to Zebra Books, 475 Park Avenue South, New York, NY. 10016. DO NOT SEND CASH!

BE CAPTIVATED BY THESE HISTORICAL ROMANCES